Mechatronics System Design in Medical Engineering

Mechatronics System Design in Medical Engineering

Guest Editors

Florin Popișter
Sergiu Dan Stan
Nikola Vitković
Milan Banić

MDPI

Basel • Beijing • Wuhan • Barcelona • Belgrade • Novi Sad • Cluj • Manchester

Guest Editors

Florin Popișter
Department of Design Engineering and Robotics
Technical University of Cluj-Napoca
Cluj-Napoca
Romania

Sergiu Dan Stan
Department of Mechatronics and Machine Dynamics
Technical University of Cluj-Napoca
Cluj-Napoca
Romani

Nikola Vitković
Faculty of Mechanical Engineering
University of Nis
Niš
Serbia

Milan Banić
Faculty of Mechanical Engineering
University of Nis
Niš
Serbia

Editorial Office
MDPI AG
Grosspeteranlage 5
4052 Basel, Switzerland

This is a reprint of the Special Issue, published open access by the journal *Applied Sciences* (ISSN 2076-3417), freely accessible at: https://www.mdpi.com/journal/applsci/special_issues/84R6B42W76.

For citation purposes, cite each article independently as indicated on the article page online and as indicated below:

Lastname, A.A.; Lastname, B.B. Article Title. *Journal Name* **Year**, *Volume Number*, Page Range.

ISBN 978-3-7258-4403-6 (Hbk)
ISBN 978-3-7258-4404-3 (PDF)
https://doi.org/10.3390/books978-3-7258-4404-3

Contents

About the Editors

Florin Popișter

Dr. Florin Popișter is an Associate Professor at the Technical University of Cluj-Napoca (UTCN), specifically in the Department of Design Engineering and Robotics. He teaches courses on the mechanical construction of industrial robots, and computer-aided design. His research revolves around cutting-edge technologies and methods in manufacturing and design engineering in areas such as: robotics; additive manufacturing; reverse engineering techniques; advanced mechanical design using CAD and finite element analysis; prototyping of mechatronic equipment; mechanical reverse engineering. His publications include work on educational collaborative robot structures and the application of AI tools in collaborative robotics. His research and teaching efforts are instrumental in driving innovation in mechanical engineering and in preparing students for the evolving landscape of Industry 4.0.

Sergiu Dan Stan

Dr. Sergiu Dan Stan is an Associate Professor in the Department of Mechatronics and Machine Dynamics at the Technical University of Cluj-Napoca, Romania, where he also earned his PhD in Mechatronics in 2007. His extensive research focuses on computer vision, parallel robots, micro- and mini-robots, the design of mechatronic systems, CAD/CAM, flexible manufacturing systems, and the mechanisms and dynamics of machines. Actively engaged in professional organizations like IEEE, ASME, EUROMECH, and IFToMM, he has contributed to numerous scientific publications and research projects, notably as a project manager and mechatronics expert for initiatives such as EMERALD, which involves 3D printing of biomimetic mechatronic systems. He has also undertaken study and documentation visits to universities in France, Italy, Germany, the USA, England, and China.

Nikola Vitković

Dr. Nikola Vitković is an Associate Professor and Head of Information System in the Faculty of Mechanical Engineering, University of Nis, Serbia. He conducted online (eLearning) and classical trainings for the public and private sectors. He has also participated in scientific and professional team projects supported by the Serbian government and industry. He participated as a researcher in the FP6, FP7, TEMPUS, ERASMUS+, and H2020 projects.

Milan Banić

Dr.-Eng. Milan Banic is an Associate Professor in the Department for Mechanical Design, Product Development and Engineering at the Faculty of Mechanical Engineering, University of Niš. His expertise encompasses mechanical design, product development, and advanced engineering analysis, with a particular focus on finite element analysis (FEA) for structural and thermal applications. Dr. Banic is also a key contributor to railway engineering, researching vehicle dynamics and obstacle detection, as well as tribology, investigating friction and wear in mechanical systems. His work extends to robotics, including the optimization of unmanned ground vehicles and high-precision drives, and the application of modern manufacturing technologies like additive manufacturing, CNC machining, and reverse engineering. Through his research and teaching, he plays a vital role in advancing mechanical engineering and preparing students for the demands of Industry 4.0.

applied sciences

MDPI

Brief Report

Exploring BiomedCLIP's Capabilities in Medical Image Analysis: A Focus on Scoliosis Detection and Severity Assessment

Bartosz Polis [1,†], Agnieszka Zawadzka-Fabijan [2,†], Robert Fabijan [3], Róża Kosińska [1], Emilia Nowosławska [1] and Artur Fabijan [1,*]

1 Department of Neurosurgery, Polish-Mother's Memorial Hospital Research Institute, 93-338 Lodz, Poland; jezza@post.pl (B.P.); roza.w.kosinska@gmail.com (R.K.); emilia.nowoslawska@iczmp.edu.pl (E.N.)
2 Department of Rehabilitation Medicine, Faculty of Health Sciences, Medical University of Lodz, 90-419 Lodz, Poland; agnieszka.zawadzka@umed.lodz.pl
3 Independent Researcher, Luton LU2 0GS, UK; robert.f.fabijan@gmail.com
* Correspondence: artur8944@wp.pl
† These authors contributed equally to this work.

Abstract: Background/Objectives: Open-source artificial intelligence models (OSAIMs), such as BiomedCLIP, hold great potential for medical image analysis. While OSAIMs are increasingly utilized for general image interpretation, their adaptation for specialized medical tasks, such as evaluating scoliosis on posturographic X-ray images, is still developing. This study aims to evaluate the effectiveness of BiomedCLIP in detecting and classifying scoliosis types (single-curve and double-curve) and in assessing scoliosis severity. Methods: The study was conducted using a dataset of 262 anonymized posturographic X-ray images from pediatric patients (ages 2–17) with diagnosed scoliosis. The images were collected between January 2021 and July 2024. Two neurosurgical experts manually analyzed the Cobb angles and scoliosis stages (mild, moderate, severe). BiomedCLIP's performance in detecting scoliosis and its type was evaluated using metrics such as accuracy, sensitivity, specificity, and AUC (Area Under the Curve). Statistical analyses, including Pearson correlation and ROC curve analysis, were applied to assess the model's performance. Results: BiomedCLIP demonstrated moderate sensitivity in detecting scoliosis, with stronger performance in severe cases (AUC = 0.87). However, its predictive accuracy was lower for mild and moderate stages (AUC = 0.75 and 0.74, respectively). The model struggled with correctly identifying single-curve scoliosis (sensitivity = 0.35, AUC = 0.53), while it performed better in recognizing double-curve cases (sensitivity = 0.78, AUC = 0.53). Overall, the model's predictions correlated moderately with observed Cobb angles (r = 0.37, $p < 0.001$). Conclusions: BiomedCLIP shows promise in identifying advanced scoliosis, but its performance is limited in early-stage detection and in distinguishing between scoliosis types, particularly single-curve scoliosis. Further model refinement and broader training datasets are essential to enhance its clinical applicability in scoliosis assessment.

Keywords: BiomedCLIP; scoliosis detection; medical image analysis; machine learning in healthcare; artificial intelligence

1. Introduction

Open-source artificial intelligence models (OSAIMs) are free, publicly available tools that have found applications in various fields, including computer science and medicine [1,2]. While OSAIMs offer advanced capabilities for processing and interpreting visual data, most of them are not specifically tailored for medical image analysis, such as X-ray images. In response to this gap, dedicated models like BiomedCLIP have been developed, combining natural language processing with medical image analysis, providing new opportunities for the evaluation and interpretation of radiological data.

The evaluation of scoliosis, a complex, three-dimensional deformity of the spinal column, traditionally relies on manual radiological interpretation by clinicians. This process includes the assessment of curvature, vertebral rotation, and spinal dynamics, typically using X-ray images in anterior–posterior (AP) and lateral views [3,4]. Identifying the degree and type of scoliosis requires significant expertise and can be time-consuming, especially when differentiating between single-curve and double-curve forms or determining the severity based on the Cobb angle [5]. Challenges such as interobserver variability and the high volume of radiological data underline the need for automated tools that could enhance accuracy and reduce workload in clinical practice. Advanced AI models, such as BiomedCLIP, offer potential solutions to these challenges by providing automated, high-sensitivity analysis tailored to medical data.

Over the past year, there has been a global increase in interest in OSAIMs. This surge in attention is partly due to the release of advanced language models such as ChatGPT, produced by OpenAI. One of OpenAI's products is Contrastive Language–Image Pretraining (CLIP), which integrates both natural language and images. This model is capable of a wide range of tasks, including zero-shot image classification, image captioning, and visual question answering [6]. CLIP achieves its remarkable results by training on a diverse dataset of images and their textual descriptions, allowing the model to learn a shared embedding space, enabling it to process and understand both text and images more efficiently.

Based on CLIP, several zero-shot models have already been developed, including medical models such as SDA-CLIP, a domain adaptation method for surgical tasks based on CLIP. It enables the recognition of surgical actions across different domains, such as virtual reality and real-life operations [7]. Another study utilizing this model was SleepCLIP, which demonstrated that CLIP could be effectively adapted to sleep staging tasks, showing potential for improving the diagnosis of sleep disorders [8].

BiomedCLIP, known in its full version as Biomed-CLIP-PubMedBERT_256-vit_base_patch16_224, is an advanced model that combines natural language processing with medical image analysis. It belongs to the category of vision–language foundation models, integrating both domains to perform complex tasks. This model was trained on a massive dataset, PMC-15M, containing 15 million "image-description" pairs from scientific articles available in PubMed Central. As a result, BiomedCLIP is capable of efficiently interpreting both medical text and images (Figure 1).

BiomedCLIP stands out due to its architecture, which combines the capabilities of PubMedBERT, a model dedicated to text analysis, with a Vision Transformer optimized for working with biomedical data. This combination allows it to achieve outstanding results across many benchmark datasets, making it one of the top models in its category.

The applications of BiomedCLIP are highly versatile. The model can be used for cross-modal retrieval (information search based on images or text), medical image classification, and answering questions related to those images. With its advanced technology, BiomedCLIP is becoming a powerful tool supporting diagnostics, scientific research, and medical education, opening new possibilities in the analysis and understanding of complex biomedical information [9].

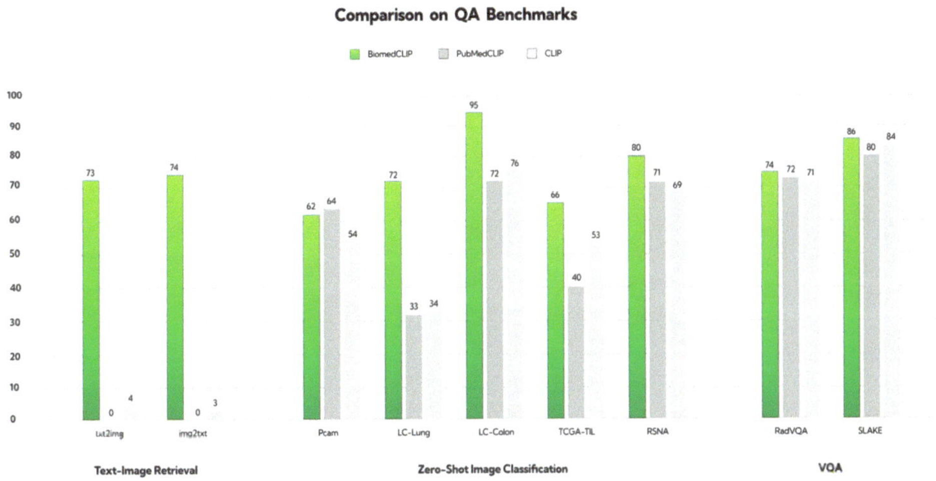

Figure 1. The creators uploaded the reconstructed figure onto the website, providing a visual representation of the performance comparison of BiomedCLIP, PubMedCLIP, and CLIP models across various QA benchmarks [9]. The results demonstrate that BiomedCLIP consistently outperforms the other models, particularly in tasks related to text-image retrieval, zero-shot image classification, and visual question answering (VQA).

Although BiomedCLIP demonstrates superior performance across most evaluated benchmarks, Figure 1 highlights an exception. In the PCam benchmark, PubMedCLIP outperformed BiomedCLIP, showcasing higher accuracy in this specific task. This observation suggests that while BiomedCLIP is a robust and versatile model, certain domain-specific datasets may still favor more specialized approaches like PubMedCLIP. This underscores the need for continued research to optimize vision–language models for diverse biomedical tasks.

Previous studies utilized the raw version of the CLIP model to evaluate posturographic X-ray images in the anteroposterior projection, demonstrating single-curve scoliosis at a severe stage. Since CLIP offers nine models with different architectures, our study partially confirmed the initial research hypothesis, indicating that only seven out of nine tested CLIP models were able to effectively recognize scoliosis from radiographic images. The second hypothesis was not confirmed, as only four of the nine models correctly answered questions regarding single-curve scoliosis. Assumptions regarding the accurate estimation of curvature degrees using AI were also not confirmed—none of the selected models achieved high sensitivity in the assessment of Cobb angles [10].

Scoliosis is a complex, three-dimensional deformity of the spinal column, identified by a curvature greater than 10 degrees, as determined by the Cobb method [11]. The diagnosis of scoliosis typically involves a comprehensive radiological posturographic examination of the entire spine in both anterior–posterior (AP) and lateral views, which facilitates the assessment of curvature, vertebral rotation, spinal dynamics, and trunk deformity, and aids in planning appropriate therapy [3,4]. Scoliosis is classified based on factors such as the patient's age, degree of curvature, underlying cause, location, and number of curves present. In this study, scoliosis is categorized into single-curve (C-shaped) and double-curve (S-shaped) forms [5]. The severity of scoliosis, as indicated by the Cobb angle, is classified into mild (10–20 degrees), moderate (20–40 degrees), and severe (greater than 40 degrees) [5,12] (Figure 2).

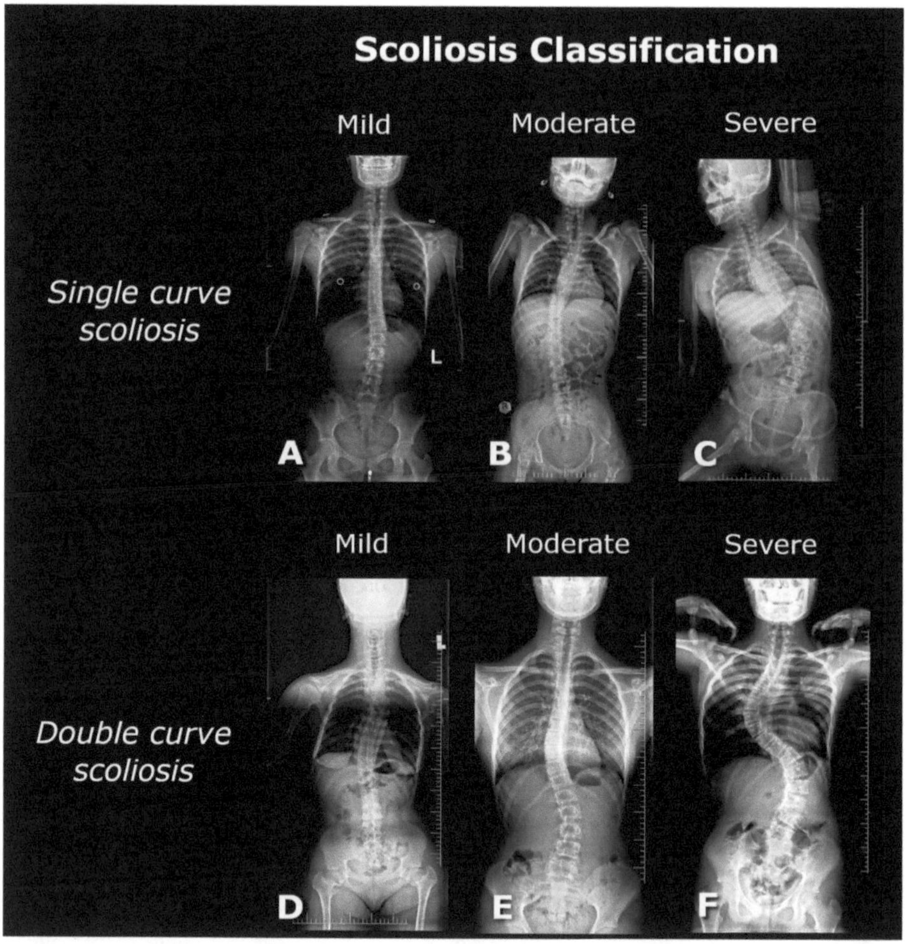

Figure 2. The figure shows posturographic X-ray images of single-curve scolioses at different stages: (**A**) mild (17° Cobb, L3/L4–Th12/Th11), (**B**) moderate (29° Cobb, L3/L4–Th7/Th6), (**C**) severe (56° Cobb, L4/L5–Th10/Th9), and double-curve scolioses: (**D**) mild (17° Cobb, L1/L2–Th9/Th8; 18° Cobb, Th8/Th7–Th2/Th1), (**E**) moderate (26° Cobb, L4/L5–L1/Th12; 25° Cobb, L1/Th12–Th8/Th7), and (**F**) severe (75° Cobb, L4/L5–Th12/Th11; 78° Cobb, Th11/Th10–Th5/Th4).

This study aimed to assess how a dedicated medical AI model, such as BiomedCLIP, performs in analyzing posturographic X-ray images that display both single-curve and double-curve scoliosis. To investigate this, three sets of questions were developed, partially building on prior research. The questions addressed whether the model detects the presence of scoliosis, correctly identifies its single-curve or double-curve form, and evaluates the severity of scoliosis—categorized as mild, moderate, or severe. Questions regarding Cobb angles were deliberately excluded, as earlier studies indicated that the CLIP model struggles with accurately determining these angles, often performing this task randomly. The following hypotheses (H) were formulated:

H1: *BiomedCLIP will detect the presence of scoliosis on all posturographic images with high sensitivity.*

H2: *BiomedCLIP will correctly identify the type of scoliosis on the provided images with high sensitivity.*

H3: *BiomedCLIP will accurately categorize the severity of scoliosis on the provided images.*

2. Materials and Methods

The study was conducted as part of the scientific research activities at the Polish-Mother's Memorial Hospital Research Institute in Poland. The bioethics committee determined that no formal consent was required for the analysis of the obtained radiological images. Posturographic images of patients diagnosed with scoliosis in the anteroposterior projection were collected between January 2021 and July 2024 (ages ranging from 2 to 17 years). Medical indications are required to perform X-ray examinations, and therefore, we did not include posturographic studies of patients without spinal deformities. Only images of patients with a prior diagnosis of scoliosis were used in this study. All images were anonymized, and consent was obtained from the legal guardians of the patients for the use of the X-ray images in this research. Inclusion criteria encompassed technically accurate images and those displaying both single-curve and double-curve scoliosis. Image quality assessment included verifying image readability and ensuring there were no errors in collimation or cropping. Exclusion criteria included scoliosis with co-occurring pathologies, such as spina bifida or vertebral hump, images that did not cover the entire spine, and scoliosis post-surgical correction with visible implants. From the X-ray image database, 262 posturographic images with visible scoliosis were included in the study. All tests were conducted using the same equipment. The X-ray images were not subjected to any modifications and were saved in JPEG format with a resolution of 2663 $\times$ 1277 px.

2.1. Manual Measurements

Analysis of the posturographic X-ray images was conducted independently by two neurosurgery specialists. RadiAnt software (version 2023.1) was used to evaluate the posturographic images.

2.2. BiomedCLIP Methodology

Model Selection and Fine-Tuning

In this study, the Biomed CLIP model was employed. This model is a fine-tuned version of the CLIP (Contrastive Language–Image Pretraining) model, specifically adapted for classifying X-ray images of children's spines into three scoliosis categories: mild, moderate, and severe. The CLIP model was selected due to its superior zero-shot classification performance and proven ability to interpret complex biomedical imagery, surpassing other multimodal models like DALL-E, MedCLIP, and PubMedCLIP. The open-source availability of the Biomed CLIP model further facilitated its use in this research.

The model was fine-tuned using the PMC-15 dataset, which includes 15 million biomedical image–text pairs derived from 4.4 million scientific articles. This broad and diverse dataset helped adapt the model to the specific demands of pediatric spinal imagery and enhanced its ability to interpret medical images.

Hyperparameters

The fine-tuning of Biomed CLIP followed the same hyperparameters as those used in training the original CLIP ViT-B/16 model (Table 1). These include:

Table 1. Hyperparameters used for fine-tuning BioMed CLIP, following the same setup as the original CLIP ViT-B/16 model.

Hyperparameter	Value
Learning Rate	4×10^{-4}
Weight Decay	0.2
Adam β1	0.9
Adam β2	0.98
Adam ε	1.00×10^{-6}
Batch Size	32,768
Training Epochs	32
Warm-up Iterations	2000
Gradient Clipping	Max temperature of 100

Hardware and Software Configuration

All computational tasks were carried out on two NVIDIA L40S GPUs, supported by 16 vCPUs and 124 GB of RAM, with 96 GB of VRAM on the RunPod platform. The software environment utilized a Docker image (pytorch:2.1.0-py3.10-cuda11.8.0-devel-ubuntu22.04) containing the necessary CUDA and PyTorch modules to support model training and evaluation.

Model Architecture

The Biomed CLIP model is based on the Vision Transformer (ViT-B/16) architecture for its vision encoder, which divides input images into 16 × 16-pixel patches. This architecture was chosen for its ability to capture long-range dependencies in medical images. Each patch is treated as a token and processed using a self-attention mechanism. The model supports images of 224 × 224 pixels, though experiments with a higher resolution (384 × 384) suggested improved performance for certain tasks, albeit with increased training time.

The ViT-B/16 model features approximately 86 million trainable parameters. To handle the specific demands of medical text, the text encoder was adjusted from the standard 77 tokens to a context size of 256 tokens, accommodating longer and more detailed biomedical descriptions.

Training Setup

Training was performed on large-scale hardware configurations using 16 NVIDIA A100 or V100 GPUs. To optimize memory usage and computational efficiency, techniques such as gradient checkpointing and automatic mixed precision were employed. The fine-tuning process was carried out for 32 epochs, with a batch size of 32,768, and the Adam optimizer was used with weight decay and a learning rate of 4×10^{-4}.

Data Handling and Evaluation

The evaluation was performed using a database of anonymized X-ray images, enabling iterative assessments of the model's classification performance across various stages of scoliosis. For this task, descriptive text labels were prepared to represent the classification of each category:

1. First Category:
    a. "This is an image of scoliosis".
    b. "This is not an image scoliosis".
2. Second Category:
    a. "This is an image of single curve scoliosis"
    b. "This is an image of double curve scoliosis"
3. Third Category:
    a. "This is an image of mild scoliosis".

b. "This is an image of moderate scoliosis".
c. "This is an image of severe scoliosis".

Each X-ray image was preprocessed through normalization before being input into the model. The model then computed the probability of the image belonging to each scoliosis category, with a confidence score ranging from 0 to 1. This score was used as a quantitative measure of the model's certainty in its predictions.

The evaluation emphasized accuracy in image classification and the ability to generalize across unseen medical image data, testing both the robustness and real-world applicability of Biomed CLIP in clinical diagnostics.

Detection and Classification Framework

Detection and Classification Methodology

Detection of Scoliosis

The detection process focused on identifying the presence of spinal deformities in posturographic X-ray images. The BiomedCLIP model was utilized to automatically determine whether a given image depicted scoliosis. The steps involved in detection included:

- **Approach**: Detection was conducted using descriptive text labels, assigning each image to one of two categories: "This is an image of scoliosis" or "This is not an image of scoliosis".
- **Parameters**:
    - The model's vision encoder, based on the ViT-B/16 architecture, divided the input images into 16 × 16-pixel patches for analysis.
    - Images were normalized and resized to 224 × 224 pixels prior to being fed into the model.
    - The text encoder was extended to handle up to 256 tokens, accommodating detailed biomedical descriptions.
- **Outcome**: The model computed the probability of the image belonging to the category of scoliosis, with confidence scores ranging from 0 to 1, providing a quantitative measure of detection.

Classification of Scoliosis

Once scoliosis was detected, the images were further classified into two additional dimensions: the type of scoliosis (single-curve or double-curve) and the severity of the condition (mild, moderate, or severe).

1. **Classification of Scoliosis Type:**
    - **Approach**: Images were categorized based on their curvature type:
        - "This is an image of single-curve scoliosis".
        - "This is an image of double-curve scoliosis".
    - **Parameters:**
        - The same preprocessing steps as in the detection process were applied, with images resized to 224 × 224 pixels and normalized.
        - Textual prompts tailored to the classification task were used to improve model specificity.
    - **Outcome**: The model assigned probabilities to each category, identifying the type of scoliosis with high confidence.
2. **Classification of Scoliosis Severity:**
    - **Approach**: Severity classification divided images into three categories:

        - Mild scoliosis ("This is an image of mild scoliosis").
        - Moderate scoliosis ("This is an image of moderate scoliosis").
        - Severe scoliosis ("This is an image of severe scoliosis").
    - **Parameters:**
        - Severity levels were defined based on the Cobb angle measurements:
            - Mild: <20°.
            - Moderate: 20°–40°.
            - Severe: >40°.
        - The model's vision encoder leveraged detailed geometric features of the X-ray images to differentiate between severity levels.
    - **Outcome**: Probabilities were calculated for each severity category, enabling precise classification of the scoliosis stage.

Integration of Detection and Classification

Both detection and classification were performed using the BiomedCLIP model, fine-tuned to handle pediatric spinal imagery. Although these processes shared a common model architecture, they were treated as distinct stages in the analysis pipeline. The detection stage established the presence of scoliosis, while the classification stages refined the analysis by identifying the specific type and severity.

By addressing detection and classification as separate processes, this methodology ensured a clear, structured workflow and optimized the model's performance for each task. The parameters and technical solutions implemented for both stages are detailed in the corresponding sections of the methodology.

2.3. Statistical Analysis

In the present analysis, the significance level was set at $\alpha = 0.05$. Descriptive statistics were employed to summarize the data. For continuous variables, the median (Mdn) served as the central tendency measure due to its robustness against outliers and distributional skewness. Furthermore, the first (Q1) and third (Q3) quartiles were reported to delineate the central 50% range of the data. Additionally, the inclusion of minimum (Min) and maximum (Max) values offers a complete view of the data's range, highlighting the extremes. Categorical variables were quantified by counts (n) and the proportion of each category. The relationship between two numerical variables was investigated using Pearson correlation. The 95% confidence intervals (CI 95%) and p-values were computed through the asymptotic approximation of the t-test statistic.

The predictive performance of the BiomedCLIP model was evaluated by determining the optimal cutpoints for dichotomous outcomes (positive class—incidence of the event, negative class—absence of the event) through a method that maximizes the sum of specificity and sensitivity. The model's discriminative ability was further assessed by estimating metrics such as accuracy, sensitivity, specificity, and the Area Under the Curve (AUC) with results visualized via Receiver Operating Characteristic (ROC) curves. To ascertain the model's predictive capability beyond mere guessing, the 95% confidence intervals for the AUC metrics were estimated employing the DeLong test [13]. A high level of sensitivity was defined as achieving a result >90%, reflecting optimal performance for early detection and classification tasks.

Specificity requires a proper equation to connect ROC, AUC, and CI calculations for single- and double-curve scoliosis.

$$Sensitivity = \frac{TP}{TP + FN}$$

$$Specificity = \frac{TN}{TN + FP},$$

where *TP*—true positive values; *FN*—false negative values; *TN*—true negative values; *FP*—false positive value.

$$AUC = \int_0^1 Sensitivity\ d(1 - Specificity),$$

where d is the difference in scores or ranks between the positive and negative classes.

Variance of AUC is defined as:

$$Var\ (AUC) = \frac{1}{n_1 n_2} \sum_{i=1}^{n1} \sum_{j=1}^{n2} (V_{ij} - AUC)^2,$$

where V_{ij} is a weight assigned to each pair of observations; n_1—number of positive instances, n_2—number of negative instances, i—index of positive instances, j—index of negative instances.

$$CI = [AUC - z \cdot SE,\ AUC + z \cdot SE],$$

where *CI*—confidence interval for AUC; *z*—is the critical value from the standard normal distribution ($z = 1.96$ for 95% confidence); *SE*—standard error, defined as:

$$SE = \sqrt{Var(AUC)}$$

Characteristics of the applied statistical tool and external packages

Analyses were conducted using the R Statistical language (version 4.3.3; [14]) on Windows 11 Pro 64 bit (build 22631), using the packages see (version 0.9.0; [15]), report (version 0.5.8; [16]), correlation (version 0.8.5; [17,18]), patchwork (version 1.2.0; [19]), pROC (version 1.18.5; [20]), gtsummary (version 1.7.2; [21]), cutpointr (version 1.1.2; [22]), ggplot2 (version 3.5.0; [23]), readxl (version 1.4.3; [24]), dplyr (version 1.1.4; [25]), and psych (version 2.4.6.26; [26]).

Characteristics of the observed data

An analysis was conducted on 262 radiographic images all identified with scoliosis. These images were assessed by two independent neurosurgical experts who evaluated the Cobb angles, scoliosis type, and its stage. The results of these assessments are presented in Table 2 and will be treated as observed data in further analyses.

Table 2. Distribution of Cobb angle measurements, types, and stages of scoliosis in a study sample of radiographic images.

Characteristic	N	n (%)
Cobb angle	262	42.00 (25.00, 66.75) [a]
Scoliosis type:	262	
Single		149 (56.87%)
Double		113 (43.13%)
Scoliosis severity:	262	
Mild		43 (16.41%)
Moderate		85 (32.44%)
Severe		134 (51.15%)

Note: [a] Mdn (Q1, Q3); N—sample size; n—group size; Mdn—median; Q1—first quartile (25%); Q3—third quartile (75%).

The examination of the data demonstrated that the median Cobb angle was 42.0 degrees, with observed values ranging from 12 to 115 degrees. The first and third quartiles were noted at 25.0 and 66.8 degrees, respectively, reflecting a significant variability in the severity of curvature across the studied sample. In terms of scoliosis type, the majority of cases were classified as single (56.87%), with double scoliosis observed in 43.13% of the samples. Regarding the staging of scoliosis, the data showed that severe scoliosis was the most common stage, accounting for 51.15% of cases, followed by moderate and mild stages at 32.44% and 16.41%, respectively.

3. Results

3.1. Analyzing the Correlation Between Observed Cobb Angles and Predictive Probabilities of Scoliosis Using the BiomedCLIP Model

The analysis utilizing the BiomedCLIP model to predict the likelihood of scoliosis from radiographic images yielded probabilities ranging from 0.097 to 0.818, demonstrating a considerable variation in the model's certainty across the spectrum of scoliosis severities and types. A correlation analysis was conducted to evaluate the relationship between the observed Cobb angles and the predictive probabilities generated by the model.

Based on the results in Table 2, in the overall sample of 262 images, a moderate correlation ($r = 0.37$) was observed, CI 95%: 0.26–0.47, which was statistically significant ($t = 6.39$, $p < 0.001$). This suggests that, generally, the model's predictions align moderately well with the clinically observed Cobb angles across all cases.

However, when the data were stratified by the stage of scoliosis, the strength of correlation varied. In the mild stage group ($n = 43$), the correlation was weaker ($r = 0.24$) and not statistically significant ($p = 0.118$), indicating a lower predictive accuracy of the model in this subgroup. The moderate stage group ($n = 85$) also showed a weaker, non-significant correlation ($r = 0.19$, $p = 0.077$). The severe stage group ($n = 134$), however, displayed a slight yet statistically significant correlation ($r = 0.18$, $p = 0.041$), suggesting some level of predictive reliability in more advanced stages of scoliosis.

The analysis within scoliosis types revealed that the model performed better in predicting the occurrence of scoliosis in both single ($r = 0.36$, $p < 0.001$) and double ($r = 0.44$, $p < 0.001$) curvature types, with both correlations being statistically significant and stronger compared to the stage-based groups. This indicates that the model is more reliable in distinguishing the type of scoliosis rather than its severity stage.

The results of the correlation analyses were depicted through scatter plots with linear regression lines, as illustrated in Figure 3.

The varying degrees of correlation across different stages and types suggest that the model's predictive capabilities may benefit from further refinement, particularly for early-stage scoliosis detection where its current predictive certainty is lower (Table 3).

Table 3. Correlation analysis between observed cobb angles and predictive probabilities of scoliosis using the BiomedCLIP model, stratified by scoliosis stage and type.

Characteristic	n_{obs}	r	CI 95%	t	p
Overall sample	262	0.37	0.26–0.47	6.39	<0.001
Within scoliosis severity forms					
Mild	43	0.24	−0.06–0.51	1.60	0.118
Moderate	85	0.19	−0.02–0.39	1.79	0.077
Severe	134	0.18	0.01–0.34	2.07	0.041
Within scoliosis types					
Single	149	0.36	0.21–0.49	4.61	<0.001
Double	113	0.44	0.28–0.58	5.23	<0.001

Note: n_{obs}—number of observations; r—Pearson's correlation coefficient; CI 95%—confidence interval 95%; t—statistic of *t*-test; *p*—*p*-value of statistical test.

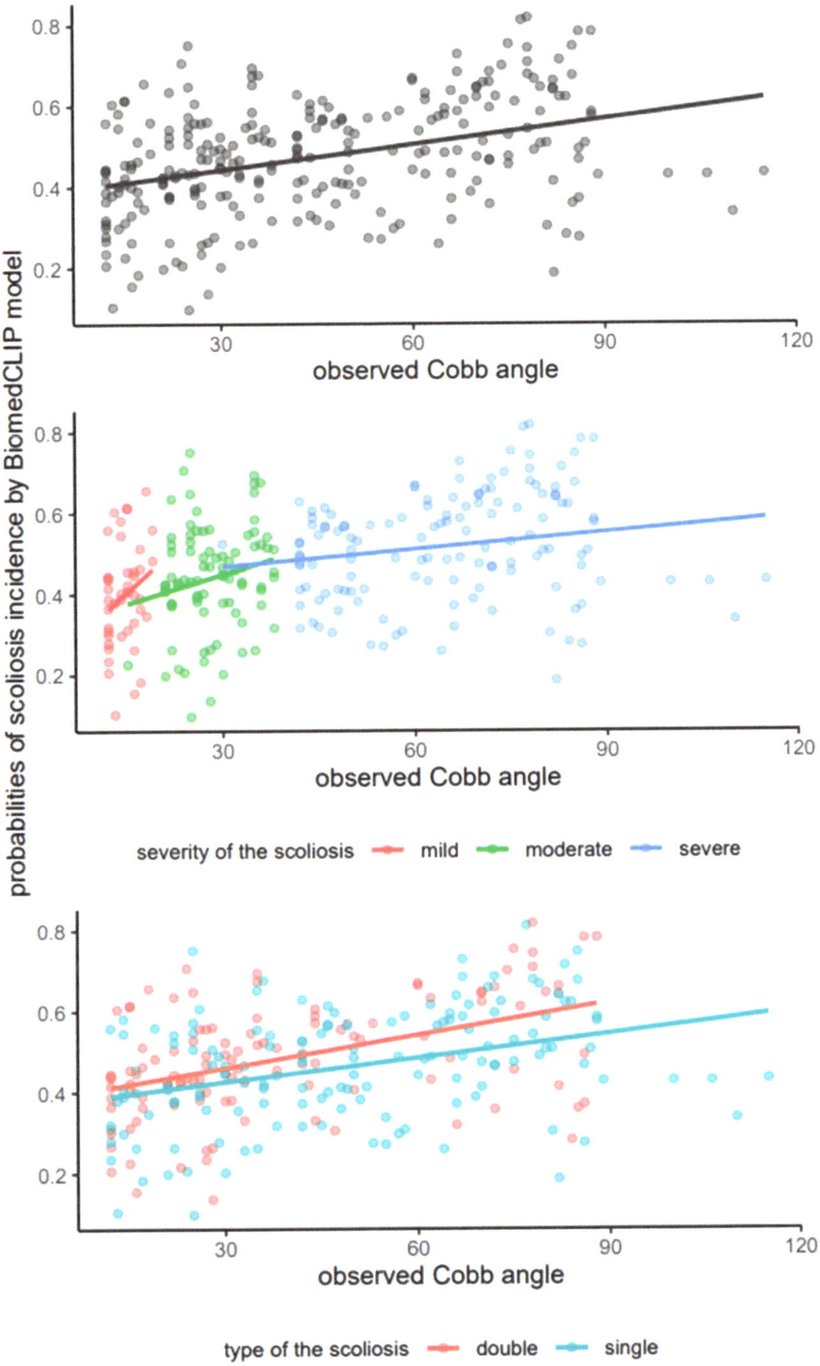

Figure 3. Scatterplots illustrating the relationship between observed Cobb angles and predicted probabilities of scoliosis incidence as determined by the BiomedCLIP model, with fitted lines for the overall sample (**upper**), scoliosis stage (**middle**), and scoliosis type (**lower**).

3.2. Estimating Optimal Cutpoints and Performance Metrics for Predictions of Scoliosis Severity and Types by BiomedCLIP Model

Analogous to the findings presented in Section 3.1, the results of the BiomedCLIP model were quantified on a numeric scale ranging from 0 to 1, representing the probability of event incidence. Descriptive statistics detailing the probabilities for events studied independently, including the occurrence of mild, moderate, and severe scoliosis, as well as single and double scoliosis types, are displayed in Table 4.

Table 4. Distribution of the probabilities of the specified event incidence by BiomedCLIP model, $N = 262$.

Characteristic	Mdn	Q1	Q3	Min	Max
		Scoliosis severity			
Mild	0.10	0.07	0.13	0.01	0.22
Moderate	0.46	0.35	0.59	0.10	0.72
Severe	0.44	0.29	0.58	0.12	0.88
		Scoliosis type			
Single curve	0.60	0.53	0.64	0.32	0.77
Double curve	0.40	0.36	0.47	0.23	0.68

Note: N—sample size; n—group size; Mdn—median; Q1—first quartile (25%); Q3—third quartile (75%), Min—minimum value; Max—maximum value.

Based in the results in Table 4, the BiomedCLIP model demonstrates differentiated predictive capabilities across different severity levels and types of scoliosis. The higher median probabilities and narrower interquartile ranges for single-curve scoliosis and moderate severity suggest that the model is more certain and consistent in these predictions. In contrast, severe scoliosis and double-curve scoliosis exhibit broader ranges of probabilities, indicating higher variability and less certainty in these predictions. This variability could stem from the inherent complexities and diverse manifestations of severe and double-curve scoliosis, which may challenge the model's predictive accuracy.

The data presented in Table 5 provide a comprehensive analysis of the BiomedCLIP model's capability to predict scoliosis severity stages and types using estimated optimal cutpoints and associated performance metrics.

Table 5. Estimated optimal cutpoints and corresponding performance metrics for the prediction of scoliosis severity stages and types via the BiomedCLIP model.

Parameter	Positive Class	Optimal Cutpoint	Accuracy	Sens.	Spec.	AUC
		Within scoliosis severity groups				
Mild	yes	≥0.10	0.64	0.79	0.61	0.75
Moderate	yes	≥0.48	0.70	0.74	0.68	0.74
Severe	yes	>0.42	0.80	0.84	0.77	0.87
		Within scoliosis types				
Single curve	yes	≥0.53	0.53	0.35	0.78	0.53
Double curve	yes	≥0.37	0.53	0.78	0.35	0.53

Note: Sens.—sensitivity; Spec.—specificity.

For the scoliosis severity forms, the model demonstrates varying degrees of effectiveness. In predicting mild scoliosis, the model achieves a moderate accuracy = 0.64, with a sensitivity = 0.79 and specificity = 0.61, supported by an AUC = 0.75, suggesting reasonable discriminative ability though with some limitations in specificity. The moderate scoliosis prediction shows a slightly better performance with an accuracy = 0.70, sensitivity = 0.74, and specificity = 0.68, which indicates a balanced ability in identifying true positives and true negatives, mirrored by an AUC = 0.74. Predictions for severe scoliosis deliver the highest accuracy = 0.80, accompanied by an impressive sensitivity = 0.84 and specificity = 0.77, reflected in the highest AUC = 0.87 among the group. This indicates a strong predictive capability of the model in identifying severe cases, which is crucial for prioritizing medical interventions. This could be attributed to more pronounced physiological markers or imaging characteristics that are easier to detect and differentiate at severe stages. The performance of the model, as visualized through ROC curves for specific scoliosis severity stages, is detailed in Figure 4. The lower boundary of the 95% confidence interval for each curve was distinctly above 0.50, indicating a clear superiority in the model's discriminative ability compared to mere guessing.

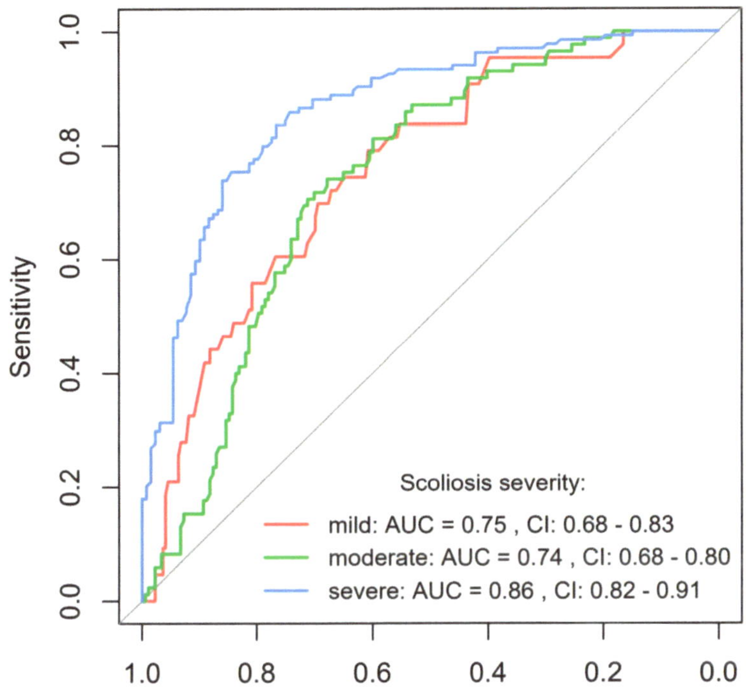

Figure 4. ROC curve analysis for scoliosis severity forms prediction using the BiomedCLIP model with AUC and 95% confidence interval.

On the other hand, the performance metrics for scoliosis types reveal a different challenge. The prediction for a single-curve-type scoliosis result in a lower accuracy = 0.53, with a notably low sensitivity = 0.35, although the specificity is relatively higher at 0.78. This indicates a significant challenge in correctly identifying cases with single-curve scoliosis, as many actual cases might go undetected. The AUC = 0.53 suggests that the model performs only slightly better than chance in this scenario. In contrast, predictions for double-curve scoliosis also show an accuracy = 0.53 but with a reversed profile of high sensitivity = 0.78 and low specificity = 0.35, resulting in an AUC = 0.53. This suggests that while the model is better at detecting the presence of double-curve scoliosis, it also misclassifies a significant number of non-double-curve cases as double-curve. The performance of the model, as visualized through ROC curves for specific scoliosis severity stages, is detailed in Figure 5. The calculated CI 95% for both curves encompassed the value of 0.50, thereby indicating that the predictive capability was no better than random guessing.

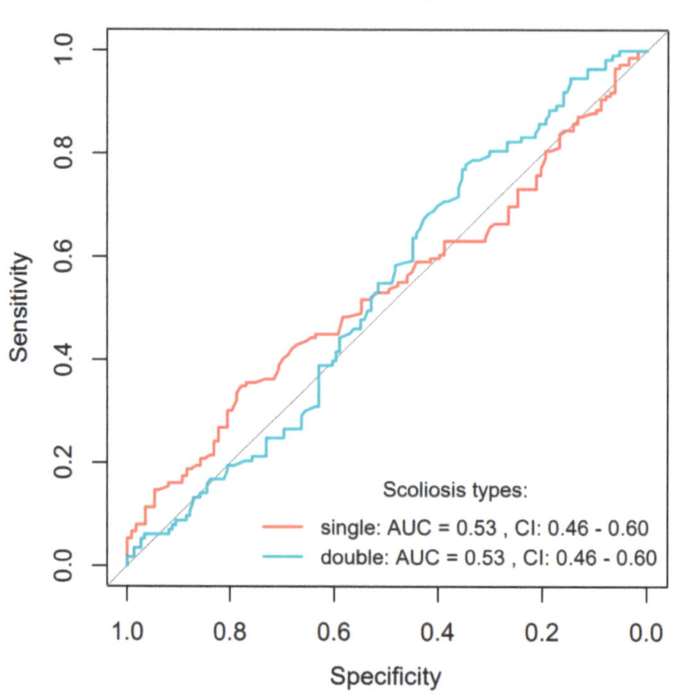

Figure 5. ROC curve analysis for scoliosis types prediction using the BiomedCLIP model with AUC and 95% confidence interval.

In conclusion, the BiomedCLIP model exhibits a robust predictive power for severe scoliosis stages, crucial for effective clinical prioritization and intervention. However, the challenges in predicting scoliosis types, particularly in distinguishing between single- and double-curve scoliosis with high accuracy and balanced sensitivity and specificity, highlight areas for potential model refinement and improvement.

4. Discussion

Our study found that the presented hypotheses regarding the effectiveness of the BiomedCLIP model in detecting scoliosis were not fully confirmed. Although the model demonstrated high sensitivity in recognizing advanced scoliosis, its effectiveness in identifying mild cases and different curvature types was limited. Particularly for single-curve scoliosis, the model's sensitivity was significantly lower than expected.

4.1. Evaluation of BiomedCLIP Sensitivity in Scoliosis Detection Across All Images

The results of the BiomedCLIP model showed an overall correlation between Cobb angles and the probabilities predicted by the model, with $r = 0.37$, indicating moderate agreement with actual clinical outcomes ($p < 0.001$). Despite statistical significance, this result does not suggest high sensitivity of the model's predictions in all cases. When analyzing differences based on scoliosis stage, the correlation in mild cases was low (r = 0.24, $p = 0.118$), indicating limited effectiveness of the model in detecting mild cases. Similarly, in the moderate stage, the correlation was weak (r = 0.19, $p = 0.077$), and in the severe stage, although statistically significant, the correlation was relatively low (r = 0.18, $p = 0.041$). These findings suggest that the model struggles to predict scoliosis in mild and moderate stages, challenging the assumption of its high sensitivity in all situations. In conclusion, Hypothesis H1 was not confirmed. The results indicate that BiomedCLIP does not achieve high sensitivity in predicting the presence of scoliosis across all posturographic images. While the model shows moderate effectiveness in more advanced cases and in predicting scoliosis types, its performance is weaker for mild and moderate stages, as well as in distinguishing scoliosis types, emphasizing the need for further optimization of the model.

The limitations in distinguishing scoliosis types highlight the necessity for improving training datasets and advanced image processing techniques to enhance the model's precision [27]. Studies suggest that the integration of diverse imaging data could enhance AI performance in clinical environments [28]. Despite these challenges, ongoing advancements in AI and imaging techniques may ultimately lead to more reliable diagnostic tools for scoliosis.

4.2. Performance of BiomedCLIP in Detecting Single-Curve and Double-Curve Scoliosis

The results of the BiomedCLIP model demonstrated limited effectiveness in predicting both single-curve and double-curve scoliosis. For single-curve scoliosis, the model achieved low accuracy (0.53) and sensitivity (0.35), indicating difficulty in detecting actual cases. Although specificity was higher (0.78), the model struggled to confirm the presence of single-curve scoliosis, with an AUC of 0.53 suggesting performance only slightly better than random guessing. For double-curve scoliosis, the model showed a reverse pattern: higher sensitivity (0.78) but low specificity (0.35), resulting in numerous false positives. Accuracy remained at 0.53, and the AUC again indicated near-random performance (0.53). These consistent AUC results underscore the model's challenges in distinguishing between single-curve and double-curve scoliosis The hypothesis (H2) that BiomedCLIP would accurately identify scoliosis types with high sensitivity was not fully confirmed. Hypothesis H2 posited that BiomedCLIP would accurately identify scoliosis types (single-curve and double-curve) with high sensitivity. However, the results demonstrated mixed outcomes. The model showed significant challenges in predicting single-curve scoliosis, achieving a sensitivity of only 0.35 and an AUC of 0.53, indicating performance slightly above random guessing. While the model exhibited higher specificity (0.78) in this category, it frequently failed to detect positive cases, leading to low overall accuracy (0.53). This suggests that the subtle radiographic features of single-curve scoliosis present a greater challenge for the model, likely due to the limited visibility of curvature in certain mild or intermediate stages. The overlapping of the two ROC curves near the middle of the sensitivity range reflects the complementary nature of the probabilities assessed by the AI model for features with two categories (single and double scoliosis). This behavior suggests that the model evaluates the features in a way that treats the two scoliosis types as interdependent or mutually exclusive.

This indicates that the AI model is likely assigning probabilities based on a shared feature set, where the sum of probabilities for both categories equals 1. The complementary probabilities reflect a balancing act by the model, where it adjusts predictions for one category as the likelihood for the other category increases. This approach is common in binary classification tasks, particularly when the model is trained on features that do not strongly distinguish between the two categories.

This complementary relationship in probability assessment is reflected in the nearly identical AUC values (0.53 for both single and double scoliosis) and the overlapping confidence intervals (CI: 0.46–0.60). These metrics suggest that the model's performance in distinguishing between the two categories is limited and heavily influenced by shared characteristics of the feature space.

In contrast, the model performed better in detecting double-curve scoliosis, achieving a sensitivity of 0.78. However, this improvement came at the cost of reduced specificity (0.35), with the model misclassifying a notable number of non-double-curve cases as positive.

The AUC value of 0.53 again highlights the lack of strong predictive capability. These results collectively suggest that while BiomedCLIP is capable of identifying double-curve scoliosis more reliably than single-curve cases, its overall performance in distinguishing scoliosis types remains limited. Further optimization, such as introducing additional training data with well-annotated examples of scoliosis types, is necessary to address these challenges. Low sensitivity for single-curve scoliosis and low specificity for double-curve scoliosis suggest that the model frequently failed to identify single-curve cases while misclassifying many as double-curve. This difficulty likely stems from the subtle imaging features of single-curve scoliosis, which are harder for the model to detect. While the model performed better in identifying double-curve scoliosis, this improvement came at the expense of increased false positives. These findings undermine the hypothesis of high sensitivity in recognizing scoliosis types and highlight the need for further optimization, particularly to improve sensitivity for single-curve scoliosis and specificity for double-curve scoliosis.

Detecting and classifying scoliosis using artificial intelligence (AI) models remains a significant challenge, especially in differentiating between these curvature types. Studies indicate that despite generally high accuracy, the sensitivity and specificity of AI models vary significantly depending on the curvature type and grade. For example, recent research demonstrated that an AI system achieved high sensitivity (0.97) and specificity (0.88) in detecting scoliosis, particularly in mild and moderate grades, while certain cases showed discrepancies exceeding 5° in Cobb angle measurement [29]. This suggests that such cases may be more difficult for models to accurately identify. While models demonstrate better sensitivity in double-curve scoliosis, this comes at the expense of an increased number of false alarms, leading to misclassification and reduced specificity [30].

These results underscore the need for further optimization of AI models to improve sensitivity in cases of single-curve scoliosis and increase specificity for double-curve scoliosis cases [31]. Techniques such as deep learning and automated ultrasound imaging are being studied to enhance diagnostic accuracy and reduce human error in measurements [31,32]. Although AI shows potential in detecting scoliosis, current limitations in sensitivity and specificity require further research and model optimization to achieve reliable clinical results.

4.3. Assessment of BiomedCLIP Accuracy in Classifying Scoliosis Severity

The results of the BiomedCLIP model in predicting scoliosis severity showed varying effectiveness depending on the disease stage. For mild scoliosis, the model achieved moderate accuracy (0.64), with a sensitivity of 0.79 and specificity of 0.61, highlighting limitations in precision. For moderate scoliosis, accuracy improved slightly to 0.70, with sensitivity at 0.74 and specificity at 0.68, indicating balanced performance in identifying true cases and reducing false positives. The best results were observed for severe scoliosis, where accuracy reached 0.80, sensitivity 0.84, and specificity 0.77, reflecting strong effectiveness in recognizing advanced cases.

The AUC analysis corroborates these findings. For mild scoliosis, the AUC was 0.75, suggesting moderate discrimination ability, while for moderate scoliosis, it was 0.74. For severe scoliosis, the AUC peaked at 0.87, underscoring excellent detection capability. The ROC curves further illustrate that the model consistently performed better than random guessing, particularly excelling in severe cases. These results indicate that BiomedCLIP performed significantly better in detecting severe scoliosis compared to mild and moderate stages. The model's stronger performance in advanced cases can be attributed to more pronounced physiological changes visible in imaging. In contrast, subtler changes in mild scoliosis presented greater challenges, especially in maintaining specificity. The difficulty in detecting mild scoliosis reflects the subtleties of the disease, which make it harder for the model to discern changes on radiographic images. Hypothesis (H3), which proposed that BiomedCLIP would accurately classify scoliosis severity, was only partially confirmed. Hypothesis H3 proposed that BiomedCLIP would accurately categorize the severity of scoliosis into mild, moderate, and severe stages. The results indicate that the model's performance varies depending on the severity stage. For severe scoliosis, BiomedCLIP achieved strong predictive power, with an accuracy of 0.80, sensitivity of 0.84, and specificity of 0.77, supported by an AUC of 0.87. These results confirm the model's robustness in detecting advanced scoliosis cases, likely due to the more pronounced radiographic markers in severe stages.

In comparison, the model's performance was more moderate for mild and moderate scoliosis. For mild cases, sensitivity reached 0.79, but accuracy was lower at 0.64, and specificity was limited to 0.61, indicating a tendency for false positives. Similarly, moderate cases showed a balanced performance with an accuracy of 0.70, sensitivity of 0.74, and specificity of 0.68, yet still fell short of the hypothesis's expectation for high predictive precision. These findings highlight that while BiomedCLIP demonstrates notable success in identifying severe scoliosis, its ability to reliably classify mild and moderate stages remains limited.

The observed variability underscores the need for further refinement of the model and expansion of training datasets. Including more annotated examples of mild and moderate scoliosis, as well as enhancing image preprocessing techniques, could improve performance across all severity stages. Advanced AI models, although promising, still face limitations in accurately assessing Cobb angles and classifying less advanced cases of scoliosis [33]. Despite these advancements, the challenges of diagnosing mild scoliosis emphasize the need for further refinement of AI models to enhance diagnostic capabilities across all severity stages.

In conclusion, the hypothesis regarding the model's ability to classify scoliosis severity was only partially confirmed. BiomedCLIP demonstrated strong performance in detecting severe scoliosis but moderate effectiveness for mild and moderate cases. Further optimization is necessary to improve detection in early and intermediate stages of scoliosis.

4.4. Comparison with CLIP

When comparing the results obtained by the CLIP and BiomedCLIP models, a key question arises: why did an untrained model like CLIP achieve 100% accuracy in detecting severe single-curve scoliosis, while BiomedCLIP, specifically trained on medical data, performed less effectively in similar cases? Notably, CLIP was tested on only 23 images of severe single-curve scoliosis, whereas BiomedCLIP analyzed a larger and more diverse dataset of 262 images, covering various severities and scoliosis types.

One explanation for this paradox is the simplicity of the task given to CLIP. Severe single-curve scoliosis presents clear and easily detectable physiological changes, enabling even an untrained model to identify these cases. The prominence of severe scoliosis in X-ray images likely made it easier for CLIP to succeed without requiring specialized medical data training. In contrast, BiomedCLIP faced a more complex task, having to differentiate not only severe scoliosis but also mild and moderate cases, as well as classify scoliosis types. This broader scope introduced additional challenges for the model.

Trained models like BiomedCLIP are also more prone to errors due to the diversity of the datasets they are trained on. Learning to recognize subtle and inconsistent nuances across a wide range of cases may dilute the model's predictive accuracy, making it less effective in straightforward tasks such as detecting severe scoliosis. This diversity, while necessary for generalization, can reduce performance when handling highly specific or obvious changes.

4.5. Model Adaptation and Generalization

Models like BiomedCLIP have shown improved performance through domain-specific adaptations, helping focus on relevant features in medical images [34]. Introducing multi-level adaptation frameworks increases the model's ability to generalize across different types of medical data, addressing domain discrepancies [35].

4.6. Challenges with False Features

Research indicates that models like CLIP can learn false correlations, reducing performance when data distribution changes [36]. Relying on such false features may limit effectiveness in scenarios with obvious but less specific changes, as the model may misinterpret signals. However, while data diversity poses challenges, it also broadens the model's learning context, potentially increasing robustness in real-world applications.

Comparing the results of CLIP and BiomedCLIP is not entirely fair, as they were tested under different conditions. CLIP was evaluated on a simple task—detecting severe single-curve scoliosis—and performed well without specialized training. BiomedCLIP, on the other hand, had to handle a wider range of cases, including differentiating scoliosis types and severities, introducing complexities that likely impacted its performance. The differing test scenarios underline that the results of these models are not directly comparable. CLIP's strong performance stemmed from a simple, focused task, while BiomedCLIP's specialization required it to navigate more challenging diagnostic cases, affecting its accuracy in severe scoliosis detection.

The performance of BiomedCLIP can also be partially attributed to limitations in the dataset used for training. The PMC-15M dataset, containing 15 million image-text pairs from PubMed Central, includes a wide variety of biomedical image types, such as microscopy and histology. However, it does not guarantee suitability for scoliosis-specific training. A 2023 PubMed search for "scoliosis" yielded only approximately 31,226 articles, representing a small fraction of the PMC database. Many of these articles may lack relevant X-ray images, focusing instead on genetic, molecular, or clinical studies. Limited access to appropriate clinical scoliosis images likely constrained BiomedCLIP's ability to detect mild cases and differentiate curvature types effectively.

BiomedCLIP's use of the ViT (Vision Transformer) architecture also presents challenges for medical data. Transformers, initially designed for large-scale text data, require extensive datasets to extract meaningful patterns. Medical data, by contrast, are often highly specialized and context-dependent. Limited, variable datasets make it difficult to identify consistent patterns, leading to potential inaccuracies in predictions. Additionally, the complexity of interpreting medical images, which often depends on expert context, adds further difficulty. These limitations underscore the need for more targeted datasets and tailored architectural adjustments to improve performance in medical imaging tasks.

A significant challenge arises from the use of contrastive learning, a major component of transformer architectures, including BiomedCLIP. Contrastive learning can exacerbate these misinterpretations, potentially leading to incorrect classifications. Moreover, the limited availability of data presents another obstacle. The creators of BiomedCLIP themselves acknowledged that small datasets are insufficient for fine-tuning models like CLIP [34]. For instance, PubMedCLIP was trained on the ROCO dataset, which contains 81,000 images [37]. However, in the case of scoliosis, there are far fewer relevant articles and even fewer high-quality, annotated scoliosis images, further restricting the available data for model training.

This leads to another issue with the PMC-15 dataset, which focuses primarily on images where the accompanying text consists mainly of annotations. These annotations can be misleading and may provide incorrect clues about the overall context. Additionally, many medical conditions require a highly specific set of parameters for diagnosis, making it difficult to classify them correctly without sufficient and accurate data. Another limitation arises from the structure of the dataset itself, which includes images and descriptions from a wide range of biomedical fields. This diversity can result in the model being overly generalized in its predictions, making it less accurate for specific conditions like scoliosis. Furthermore, the lack of open-access PubMed articles restricts access to complete imaging datasets, which may have affected the quality and diversity of the training data available for BiomedCLIP. It is also important to note that our analysis was limited to radiographic images, which could restrict the generalizability of the results to other imaging techniques, such as MRI or CT. The lack of relevant data from other biomedical imaging modalities may have further constrained the model's effectiveness in the broader diagnostic context of scoliosis.

Recent advancements in deep learning (DL) have significantly improved scoliosis detection and quantification, particularly in tasks such as axial vertebral rotation (AVR) estimation and Cobb angle (CA) measurement. For example, Zhao et al. proposed an automatic AVR measurement method that combines vertebra landmark detection and pedicle segmentation using an improved High-Resolution Network (HR-Net) with CoordConv layers and self-attention mechanisms. Their approach demonstrated high accuracy in estimating AVR by precisely extracting pedicle center coordinates and vertebral landmarks. This landmark-based approach provides detailed structural information, which is critical for assessing three-dimensional spinal deformities, particularly in adolescent idiopathic scoliosis (AIS) [38].

Similarly, a recent systematic review of DL methods for CA measurement highlights various approaches, such as U-Net variants, Capsule Neural Networks (CapsNets), and multi-stage pipelines, achieving notable accuracy in estimating spinal curvature. For instance, CapsNet achieved a Pearson correlation coefficient (PCC) of 0.93, while LocNet and RegNet models demonstrated robust vertebral localization and CA prediction performance. These approaches rely on precise manual annotations of vertebral landmarks and demonstrate strong capabilities in quantifying curvature, which remains a gold standard for scoliosis severity assessment [39].

Our study differs from these methods by addressing scoliosis classification tasks, specifically severity stages (mild, moderate, severe) and curvature types (single-curve, double-curve), using the BiomedCLIP model. Unlike landmark-dependent AVR or CA measurement methods, BiomedCLIP leverages a contrastive learning framework to embed image–text relationships, enabling classification without requiring explicit anatomical markers or angle calculations. This approach is particularly advantageous for automating scoliosis triage and broad classification in clinical settings.

However, similar challenges are observed across studies, including our own. While AVR- and CA-based methods achieve high precision in quantifying spinal deformities, they often require extensive manual annotations and are sensitive to image quality and data variability. Our findings, such as the lower sensitivity for mild scoliosis and reduced specificity for double-curve detection, align with these limitations. Moreover, subtle imaging features in early-stage scoliosis remain a significant challenge for both CA-based measurement and classification approaches.

Integrating precise AVR and CA measurement techniques with models like BiomedCLIP represents a promising direction for future research. By combining detailed anatomical quantification with classification-based predictions, a more comprehensive AI-driven framework could be developed, enhancing scoliosis diagnosis, severity assessment, and treatment planning.

This suggests the need for further optimization of the model, as discussed earlier, to improve its sensitivity in detecting subtle cases of scoliosis and accurately differentiate curvature types. Integrating precise AVR and CA estimation techniques with BiomedCLIP's classification framework could be a valuable direction for future research.

5. Conclusions

Our study found that the initial hypotheses regarding the performance of the Biomed-CLIP model in detecting scoliosis were not fully confirmed. While the model showed high sensitivity in recognizing advanced scoliosis, its effectiveness in identifying mild cases and different types of scoliosis was limited, particularly in detecting single-curve scoliosis.

BiomedCLIP performed well in classifying advanced scoliosis, but struggled with early-stage detection and distinguishing between different types of scoliosis, especially when compared to previous results with CLIP models. Though BiomedCLIP demonstrated better differentiation of scoliosis severity, its accuracy in detecting specific types of scoliosis remained inconsistent.

In conclusion, BiomedCLIP excelled in detecting advanced scoliosis but requires further refinement to improve its performance in early-stage detection and in distinguishing between different scoliosis types. Further optimization and broader data training will be essential to enhance the model's overall accuracy and clinical applicability.

Author Contributions: Conceptualization, A.F., R.F. and A.Z.-F.; methodology, A.F., R.F., A.Z.-F. and B.P.; investigation, A.F., B.P., A.Z.-F. and R.F.; data curation, A.F., R.K. and B.P.; writing—original draft preparation, A.F., A.Z.-F., B.P., R.K. and R.F.; writing—review and editing, A.F., A.Z.-F., R.F., B.P., R.K. and E.N.; supervision, B.P. and E.N.; funding acquisition, A.F., E.N. and B.P. All authors have read and agreed to the published version of the manuscript.

Funding: This research received no external funding.

Institutional Review Board Statement: Not applicable.

Informed Consent Statement: Not applicable.

Data Availability Statement: The data are contained within the article.

Acknowledgments: Many thanks are extended to Agnieszka Strzała for linguistic proofreading and to Robert Fabijan for the substantive support in the field of AI and for assistance in designing the presented study.

Conflicts of Interest: The authors declare no conflicts of interest.

References

1. Daeschler, S.C.; Bourget, M.H.; Derakhshan, D.; Sharma, V.; Asenov, S.I.; Gordon, T.; Cohen-Adad, J.; Borschel, G.H. Rapid automated nerve histomorphometry through open-source artificial intelligence. *Sci. Rep.* **2022**, *12*, 5975. [CrossRef] [PubMed]
2. Hentschel, S.; Kobs, K.; Hotho, A. CLIP knows image aesthetics. *Front. Artif. Intell.* **2022**, *5*, 976235. [CrossRef] [PubMed]
3. Yang, F.; He, Y.; Deng, Z.S.; Yan, A. Improvement of automated image stitching system for DR X-ray images. *Comput. Biol. Med.* **2016**, *71*, 108–114. [CrossRef] [PubMed]
4. Hwang, Y.S.; Lai, P.L.; Tsai, H.Y.; Kung, Y.C.; Lin, Y.Y.; He, R.J.; Wu, C.T. Radiation dose for pediatric scoliosis patients undergoing whole spine radiography: Effect of the radiographic length in an auto-stitching digital radiography system. *Eur. J. Radiol.* **2018**, *108*, 99–106. [CrossRef]
5. Hey, H.W.D.; Ramos, M.R.D.; Lau, E.T.; Tan, J.H.J.; Tay, H.W.; Liu, G.; Wong, H.K. Risk Factors Predicting C- Versus S-shaped Sagittal Spine Profiles in Natural, Relaxed Sitting: An Important Aspect in Spinal Realignment Surgery. *Spine* **2020**, *45*, 1704–1712 [CrossRef]
6. OpenAI. CLIP: Connecting Text and Images. Available online: https://openai.com/research/clip (accessed on 29 July 2024).

7. Li, Y.; Jia, S.; Song, G.; Wang, P.; Jia, F. SDA-CLIP: Surgical visual domain adaptation using video and text labels. *Quant. Imaging Med. Surg.* **2023**, *13*, 6989–7001. [CrossRef]
8. Yang, W.; Wang, Y.; Hu, J.; Yuan, T. Sleep CLIP: A Multimodal Sleep Staging Model Based on Sleep Signals and Sleep Staging Labels. *Sensors* **2023**, *23*, 7341. [CrossRef]
9. BiomedCLIP-PubMedBERT_256-Vit_Base_Patch16_224. Available online: https://huggingface.co/microsoft/BiomedCLIP-PubMedBERT_256-vit_base_patch16_224 (accessed on 2 September 2024).
10. Fabijan, A.; Fabijan, R.; Zawadzka-Fabijan, A.; Nowosławska, E.; Zakrzewski, K.; Polis, B. Evaluating Scoliosis Severity Based on Posturographic X-ray Images Using a Contrastive Language–Image Pretraining Model. *Diagnostics* **2023**, *13*, 2142. [CrossRef]
11. Maharathi, S.; Iyengar, R.; Chandrasekhar, P. Biomechanically designed Curve Specific Corrective Exercise for Adolescent Idiopathic Scoliosis gives significant outcomes in an Adult: A case report. *Front. Rehabil. Sci.* **2023**, *4*, 1127222. [CrossRef]
12. Horng, M.H.; Kuok, C.P.; Fu, M.J.; Lin, C.J.; Sun, Y.N. Cobb Angle Measurement of Spine from X-Ray Images Using Convolutional Neural Network. *Comput. Math. Methods Med.* **2019**, *2019*, 6357171. [CrossRef]
13. DeLong, E.R.; DeLong, D.M.; Clarke-Pearson, D.L. Comparing the areas under two or more correlated receiver operating characteristic curves: A nonparametric approach. *Biometrics* **1988**, *44*, 837–845. [CrossRef] [PubMed]
14. R Core Team. *R: A Language and Environment for Statistical Computing*; R Foundation for Statistical Computing: Vienna, Austria, 2021; Available online: https://www.R-project.org/ (accessed on 2 September 2024).
15. Lüdecke, D.; Patil, I.; Ben-Shachar, M.; Wiernik, B.; Waggoner, P.; Makowski, D. see: An R Package for Visualizing Statistical Models. *J. Open Source Softw.* **2021**, *6*, 3393. [CrossRef]
16. Makowski, D.; Lüdecke, D.; Patil, I.; Thériault, R.; Ben-Shachar, M.; Wiernik, B. Automated Results Reporting as a Practical Tool to Improve Reproducibility and Methodological Best Practices Adoption. CRAN 2023. Available online: https://easystats.github.io/report/ (accessed on 2 September 2024).
17. Makowski, D.; Wiernik, B.; Patil, I.; Lüdecke, D.; Ben-Shachar, M. Correlation: Methods for Correlation Analysis. Version 0.8.3. 2022. Available online: https://CRAN.R-project.org/package=correlation (accessed on 2 September 2024).
18. Makowski, D.; Ben-Shachar, M.; Patil, I.; Lüdecke, D. Methods and Algorithms for Correlation Analysis in R. *J. Open Source Softw.* **2020**, *5*, 2306. [CrossRef]
19. Pedersen, T. Patchwork: The Composer of Plots. R Package Version 1.2.0. 2024. Available online: https://CRAN.R-project.org/package=patchwork (accessed on 2 September 2024).
20. Robin, X.; Turck, N.; Hainard, A.; Tiberti, N.; Lisacek, F.; Sanchez, J.; Müller, M. pROC: An open-source package for R and S+ to analyze and compare ROC curves. *BMC Bioinform.* **2011**, *12*, 77. [CrossRef]
21. Sjoberg, D.; Whiting, K.; Curry, M.; Lavery, J.; Larmarange, J. Reproducible Summary Tables with the gtsummary Package. *R. J.* **2021**, *13*, 570–580. [CrossRef]
22. Thiele, C.; Hirschfeld, G. cutpointr: Improved Estimation and Validation of Optimal Cutpoints in R. *J. Stat. Softw.* **2021**, *98*, 1–27. [CrossRef]
23. Wickham, H. *Ggplot2: Elegant Graphics for Data Analysis*; Springer: New York, NY, USA, 2016; ISBN 978-3-319-24277-4.
24. Wickham, H.; Bryan, J. Readxl: Read Excel Files. R Package Version 1.4.3. 2023. Available online: https://CRAN.R-project.org/package=readxl (accessed on 2 September 2024).
25. Wickham, H.; François, R.; Henry, L.; Müller, K.; Vaughan, D. Dplyr: A Grammar of Data Manipulation. R Package Version 1.1.2. 2023. Available online: https://CRAN.R-project.org/package=dplyr (accessed on 2 September 2024).
26. Revelle, W. *Psych: Procedures for Psychological, Psychometric, and Personality Research, R Package Version 2.3.9*; Northwestern University: Evanston, IL, USA, 2023. Available online: https://CRAN.R-project.org/package=psych (accessed on 2 September 2024).
27. Fabijan, A.; Zawadzka-Fabijan, A.; Fabijan, R.; Zakrzewski, K.; Nowosławska, E.; Po-lis, B. Assessing the Accuracy of Artificial Intelligence Models in Scoliosis Classification and Suggested Therapeutic Approaches. *J. Clin. Med.* **2024**, *13*, 4013. [CrossRef]
28. Maaliw, R.R.; Susa, J.A.B.; Alon, A.S.; Lagman, A.C.; Ambat, S.C.; Garcia, M.B.; Piad, K.C.; Raguro, M.C.F. A Deep Learning Approach for Automatic Scoliosis Cobb Angle Identification. In Proceedings of the 2022 IEEE World AI IoT Congress (AIIoT), Seattle, WA, USA, 6–9 June 2022; pp. 111–117. [CrossRef]
29. Kassab, D.K.I.; Kamyshanskaya, I.G.; Trukhan, S.V. A new artificial intelligence program for the automatic evaluation of scoliosis on frontal spinal radiographs: Accuracy, advantages and limitations. *Digit. Diagn.* **2024**, *5*, 243–254. [CrossRef]
30. Xie, K.; Lei, W.; Zhu, S.; Chen, Y.; Lin, J.; Li, Y.; Yan, Y. Application of Deep Learning to Diagnose and Classify Adolescent Idiopathic Scoliosis. *Chin. J. Med. Instrum.* **2024**, *48*, 126–131. [CrossRef]
31. Banerjee, S.; Huang, Z.; Lyu, J.; Leung, F.H.F.; Lee, T.; Yang, D.; Zheng, Y.; McAviney, J.; Ling, S.H. Automatic Assessment of Ultrasound Curvature Angle for Scoliosis Detection Using 3-D Ultrasound Volume Projection Imaging. *Ultrasound Med. Biol.* **2024**, *50*, 647–660. [CrossRef]
32. Gardner, A.; Berryman, F.; Pynsent, P. How Accurate are Anatomical Surface Topography Parameters in Indicating the Presence of a Scoliosis? *Spine* **2024**, *49*, 1645–1651. [CrossRef] [PubMed]

33. Fabijan, A.; Zawadzka-Fabijan, A.; Fabijan, R.; Zakrzewski, K.; Nowosławska, E.; Polis, B. Artificial Intelligence in Medica Imaging: Analyzing the Performance of ChatGPT and Microsoft Bing in Scoliosis Detection and Cobb Angle Assessmen *Diagnostics* **2024**, *14*, 773. [CrossRef] [PubMed]
34. Zhang, S.; Xu, Y.; Usuyama, N.; Xu, H.; Bagga, J.; Tinn, R.; Preston, S.; Rao, R.; Wei, M.; Valluri, N.; et al. BiomedCLIP: A multimodal biomedical foundation model pretrained from fifteen million scientific image-text pairs. *arXiv* **2023**, arXiv:2303.00915
35. Huang, C.; Jiang, A.; Feng, J.; Zhang, Y.; Wang, X.; Wang, Y. Adapting Visual-Language Models for Generalizable Anomaly Detec-tion in Medical Images. *arXiv* **2024**, arXiv:2403.12570. [CrossRef]
36. Wang, Q.; Lin, Y.; Chen, Y.; Schmidt, L.; Han, B.; Zhang, T. Do CLIPs Always Generalize Better than ImageNet Models? *arXiv* **2024**, arXiv:2403.11497. [CrossRef]
37. Pelka, O.; Koitka, S.; Rückert, J.; Nensa, F.; Friedrich, C.M. Radiology Objects in COntext (ROCO): A Multimodal Image Dataset. In *Intravascular Imaging and Computer Assisted Stenting and Large-Scale Annotation of Biomedical Data and Expert Label Synthesis*; Stoyanov, D., Taylor, Z., Balocco, S., Sznitman, R., Martel, A., Maier-Hein, L., Duong, L., Zahnd, G., Demirci, S. Albarqouni, S., et al., Eds.; LABELS CVII STENT 2018; Lecture Notes in Computer Science; Springer: Cham, Switzerland, 2018 p. 11043. [CrossRef]
38. Zhao, Y.; Zhang, J.; Li, H.; Wang, Q. Automatic axial vertebral rotation estimation on radiographs for adolescent idiopathic scoliosis by deep learning. *Biomed. Signal Process. Control.* **2024**, *88*, 105711. [CrossRef]
39. Kumar, R.; Gupta, M.; Abraham, A. A Critical Analysis on Vertebra Identification and Cobb Angle Estimation Using Deep Learning for Scoliosis Detection. *IEEE Access* **2024**, *12*, 11170–11184. [CrossRef]

applied sciences

MDPI

Article

Comparative Study Using CAD Optimization Tools for the Workspace of a 6DOF Parallel Kinematics Machine

Sergiu-Dan Stan [1], Florin Popişter [2,*], Alexandru Oarcea [1,*] and Paul Ciudin [2]

1 Department of Mechatronics and Machine Dynamics, Faculty of Automotive, Mechatronics and Mechanical Engineering, Technical University of Cluj-Napoca, B-dul Muncii 103–105, 400641 Cluj-Napoca, Romania
2 Department of Design Engineering and Robotics, Faculty of Industrial Engineering, Robotics and Production Management, Technical University of Cluj-Napoca, B-dul Muncii 103–105, 400641 Cluj-Napoca, Romania
* Correspondence: florin.popister@muri.utcluj.ro (F.P.); alexandru.oarcea@mdm.utcluj.ro (A.O.)

Abstract: This paper deals with an up-to-date topic among robotic industrial applications that require a high degree of speed, rigidity, and orientation. Currently, when technology and software applications reach a high level of performance, in various robotic industrial applications that start from certain concepts, the implementation of efficient structures has proven to be challenging. New structures such as the parallel kinematic machine (PKM) category has proven its efficiency through its structure in terms of high inertia rigidity and high speeds during processes. This paper deals with the subject of PKM-type structures in terms of the optimal design workspace of such a structure. The calculation of the workspace is considered the premise from which it starts in terms of its implementation in a robotic production line. The entire process of calculating the workspace for a given PKM structure is carried out through modern CAD applications that have specific modules in place in this direction. CATIA V5 offers the possibility through the product engineering optimizer module, simulation and calculation of different scenarios aimed at identifying the volume of the workspace for a PKM structure. In the article, we demonstrate the relations between the robot workspace and the design parameters, a method that can also be applied for other parallel structures. The method is useful for robot designers in the optimization of parallel robots with regard to the workspace by using CAD tools. Previous research in the field refers of the usage of CAD tools only for visual representation and not for optimizing the workspace, while this study and test results show that CAD tools are suitable for analyzing and optimizing the robot workspace of the 6DOF parallel robot, due to its easiness in application and fast implementation time.

Keywords: PKM; workspace; CAD; 6DOF; simulated annealing; optimal design

1. Introduction

The scope of the current paper is to apply advanced CAD (computer-aided design) knowledge within dedicated modules, using specific tools for simulation and calculus oriented on workspace capabilities and other aspects related to the robots having PKM (parallel kinematics machines) structures. Modern manufacturing systems, in means of structures, are designed with the aim of changing their usage domain using interchangeable end effectors. Ref. [1] underlines that before implantation, all aspects regarding processes or product validation undergo tests through simulations using digital manufacturing. In many industrial applications where robotic structures are involved, characteristics regarding the ability to change position and orientation with a high precision ability are a fundamental requisite. It is known that all these robotic tasks are performed with a limitation in terms of the range of rotation or even the workspace volume [2]. Adequate equipment meets the requirements by simply making precise movements within their range of six degrees of freedom. For the first time, as it is presented in the literature, these parallel kinematics machines were used in the aircraft industry in the tires test [3–6]. In terms of the practical applications within different industries where implemented parallel robotic architectures can be found, the following tools can be underlined: parallel machine tools [7], vibration simulators with six DOF (degrees of freedom) [8] and/or motion simulators [9].

One of the key challenges within these novel PKM structures are related to their capabilities regarding the workspace. Workspace analysis of a parallel kinematic machine (PKM) using tools from a CAD optimization software offers the possibility to identify the movements, volume, and trajectories. It also indicates if there are any problems due to kinematics that need to be calculated or identified, regarding the parallel robots' structures that focus on inverse or forward kinematics [6]. In the article, the relations between the robot workspace and the design parameters are demonstrated, a method that can be applied for other parallel structures as well. The method is useful for robot designers in the optimization of parallel robots with regard to the workspace by using CAD tools. Previous research in the field refers of the usage of CAD tools only for visual representation and not for optimizing the workspace [10], while this study and test results show that CAD tools are suitable for analyzing and optimizing the robot workspace of the 6DOF parallel robots, due to its easiness in application and fast implementation time.

The present work is focused on the functional design of a parallel kinematic machine (PKM) with six degrees of freedom (DOF). We studied and presented the aspects regarding the workspace determination via CAD techniques as well as numerical techniques.

The present study deals with the aspects mentioned above and starts with the theoretical side that is realized in the digital CAD space, before moving to the validation area by comparison with the analytical calculation level. The motivation for this research was to develop a novel PKM structure that has six DOF capable of adapting to different types of assembly process in a manufacturing plant.

2. Theoretical Aspects

2.1. Workspace Analysis Using Computer-Aided Design Applied for Parallel Kinematic Machines

Any additional study concerning the movement behavior of the robot regarding a desired job must first determine the workspace for any moving structure. Geometrical, numerical, and analytical methodologies may all be used to establish the workspace, and each method has its own set of benefits and drawbacks depending on the required workspace parameters [10].

Each technique for determining the workspace may be achieved in a variety of methods, and depending on the implementation and accuracy aspects, some approaches are easier to achieve than others. The geometrical technique entails creating the workspace volume by intersecting each kinematic chain of the PKM, resulting in the workspace volume of the PKM's whole structure [11]. This method is simple to perform using CAD software and CAD tools, and it generates a model of the entire theoretical workspace [12,13]. One disadvantage with using this approach in the case of PKM is that some construction factors, such as limit angles for revolute joints, can be difficult to execute, and in most PKM, the moving platform, which closes all the kinematic chains, is difficult to create independently from the kinematic chains [13,14].

2.2. The Ability to Use Multiple Types of Algorithms Using Optimization Tools from CATIA V5

Modern computer-aided design programs offer multiple numerical calculation possibilities. We can use these algorithms to calculate different optimization methods, such as minimization, maximization or even target value. In the current study, we use the CAD system CATIA V5 to maximize the workspace volume of the PKM structure. The following list introduces the possible algorithms that can be implemented:

- Simulated annealing is a random-search technique, which was developed in 1983 to deal with highly nonlinear problems. The ability to avoid being stuck in local minima is SA's main advantage over other approaches. The algorithm uses a random search, which accepts both modifications that decrease and some changes that enhance the objective function [13,14].

- For the gradient algorithm without constraints, the geometry is modified to improve its performance. Considering all the factors, it is necessary to determine the variable denoted shape sensitivity of the objective function with reference to the CAD parameters [13,14].
- The algorithm for constraints and derivative providers implements a technique for determining a viable route along which the desired function is substantially reduced. The method performs a reasonably large step length along the desired direction and utilizes the information on the optimal solution gained during the algorithm's iterations [14].
- The gradient algorithm with constraints searches for options on a local level. It works with non-essential conditions, or those whose failure does not cause the issue of inadequacy. Constraints are often broken during the optimization algorithm in this approach [15].
- The improved harmony search method with global sharing factors based on natural number coding, the multi-objective method based on the adaptive harmony search algorithm with simulation and creation and the swarm intelligence optimization algorithm [16–18].

2.3. Presentation of the PKM Structure

The mechanical structure model was designed and created in CATIA V5 according to the kinematic scheme of the robot structure illustrated in Figure 1. Stiffness, accuracy, and other performance characteristics were used to develop the robotic manipulator. Because workspace determines the extent to which a robot may be used, it is a crucial concern in the design process [16,17,19,20]. In Figure 2, the 3D model of the PKM structure is displayed.

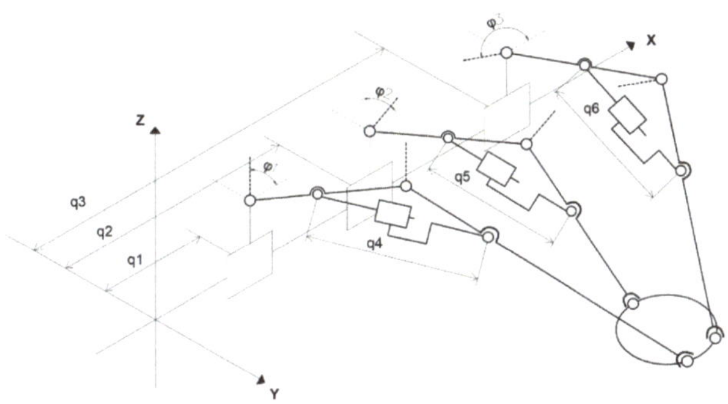

Figure 1. The kinematic scheme of the 6DOF PKM structure.

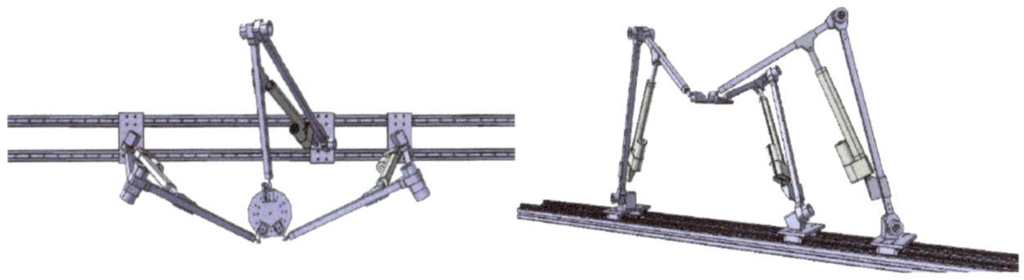

Figure 2. Views of the CAD model of the 6DOF PKM structure.

Increasing the workspace volume expands the robot's capabilities by modifying the geometrical structure. The volume and form of the workspace are influenced by several geometrical design parameters, which are presented in Table 1. The product engineering optimizer module from Dassault Systems CATIA V5 seeks to maximize the workspace volume based on the constrained parameters.

Table 1. PKM structure configuration parameters.

Parameter	Value
φ1	60°
φ2	60°
φ3	60°
d	90 mm
link1	684 mm
link2	492.75 mm
r1	397.5 mm
r2	1172.5 mm

3. Investigation of the Workspace Volume

The major interest in the determination of the workspace volume through analytic methods is associated with the involvement of each construction parameter of the PKM structure and the analysis of the behavior of each parameter to determine if optimal singular solutions exist and if they can be determined based on multiple requirements, such as imposed workspace volume, imposed inscribed workspace volume or geometric constraints.

3.1. Analytic Determination of the PKM Workspace Volume

Considering the kinematic structure of the six DOF PKM, the three $\underline{P}$R(R$\underline{P}$R)RS share predefined support planes. The actuated (R$\underline{P}$R) kinematic chain from the $\underline{P}$R(R$\underline{P}$R)RS kinematic chain imposes a fixed radius between the last joint of the chain, the spherical joint S, and the first revolute joint R of the chain. Depending on the total stroke of the actuated prismatic joint P from the (R$\underline{P}$R) chain, a minimal and maximal radius are obtained, meaning that the $\underline{P}$R(R$\underline{P}$R)RS chain has a circular workspace, as shown in Figure 3, inside the support plane, centered in the revolute center of the first revolute joint R [20].

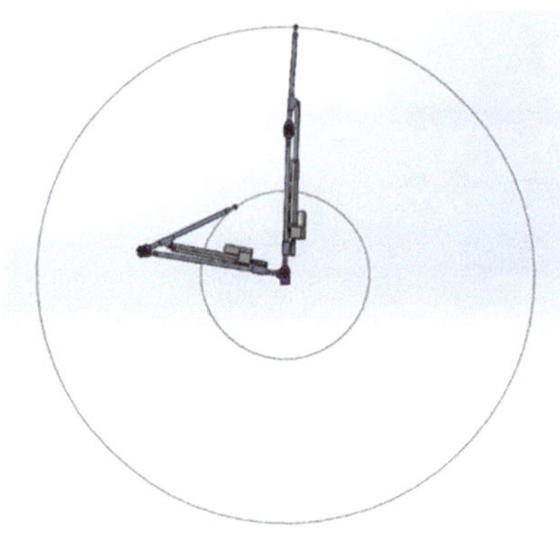

Figure 3. Representation of the workspace of each $\underline{P}$R(R$\underline{P}$R)RS upper view.

Given the fact that each of the three $\underline{P}$R(R$\underline{P}$R)RS kinematic chains defines an individual support plane that is actuated by the first prismatic joints of the previously mentioned kinematic chains, the workspace of the PKM structure is generated by translating the resulting section, as shown in Figure 4, among the prismatic axes.

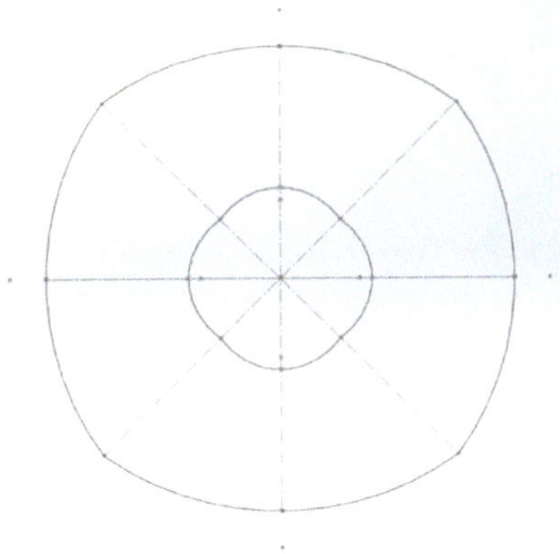

Figure 4. Representation of the resulting section of the workspace.

The resulting section of the workspace is constructed by the intersection of four curves, as shown in Figure 5, which resulted from the projection on the normal plane to the prismatic axis of the workspaces of the three PR(RPR)RS kinematic chains. The resulting shape is constructed on the intersection of only four ellipses by considering the symmetry of the structure that has the same tilt angle for the support plane of the first and last PR(RPR)RS kinematic chains.

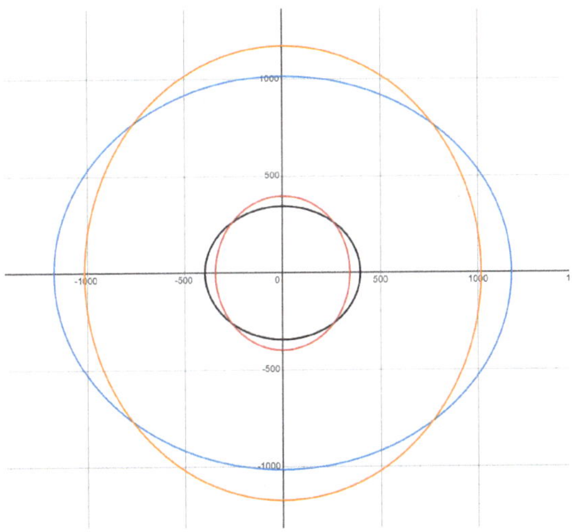

Figure 5. Representation of the four ellipses used to construct the section of the workspace (e_1—red, e_2—orange, e_3—black, e_4—blue).

The four ellipses that determine the section are as follows:

$$e_1 : \frac{y^2}{R_1^2 \cdot \sin(\varphi_1)^2} + \frac{z^2}{R_1^2} = 1 \tag{1}$$

$$e_2 : \frac{y^2}{R_2^2 \cdot \sin(\varphi_1)^2} + \frac{z^2}{R_2^2} = 1 \tag{2}$$

$$e_3: \frac{y^2}{R_1^2} + \frac{z^2}{R_1^2 \cdot \sin(\varphi_2)^2} = 1 \quad (3)$$

$$e_4: \frac{y^2}{R_2^2} + \frac{z^2}{R_2^2 \cdot \sin(\varphi_2)^2} = 1 \quad (4)$$

where

- R_1 and R_2 are the minimal and maximal radiuses imposed by the (RPR) chains for the PR(RPR)RS chains;
- φ_1 is the tilt angle of the first and last support plane;
- φ_2 is the tilt angle of the second support plane.

For the determination of the workspace volume, it is required to determine the area of the cross section of the workspace. Considering that the section of the workspace is constructed by the intersection of four ellipses centered in the same point, the resulting geometrical shape for the section of the workspace has two-fold symmetry among the major axis of the coordinate system (OY and OZ). In the case in which the values for the tilt angles φ_1, φ_2 and φ_3 are equal, the cross section gains symmetry, as shown in Figure 6, among the four major axes (OY, OZ, axis Y = Z and axis Y = −Z).

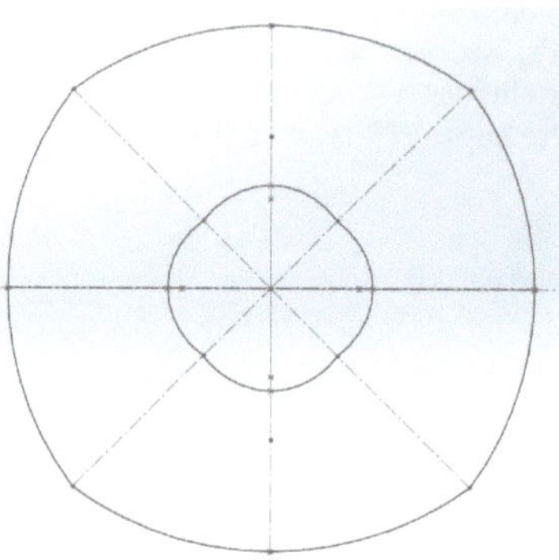

Figure 6. Representation of the two-fold symmetry of the cross section.

Considering the symmetries of the cross section, the determination of the area of the cross section for the reachable workspace, as shown in Figure 7, was implemented by using the formula for the area of an ellipse sector.

In this case, the area of the shaded region from the previous figure is as follows:

$$A = \frac{\pi \cdot R_2^2 \cdot \sin(\varphi_1)}{2} - R_2^2 \cdot \sin(\varphi_1) \cdot \text{atan}\left(\frac{\tan(\alpha)}{\sin(\varphi_1)}\right) - R_1^2 \cdot \sin(\varphi_2) \cdot \text{atan}\left(\frac{\tan(\alpha)}{\sin(\varphi_2)}\right) \quad (5)$$

$$A = R_2^2 \cdot \sin(\varphi_1) \cdot \left(\frac{\pi}{2} - \text{atan}\left(\frac{\tan(\alpha)}{\sin(\varphi_1)}\right)\right) - R_1^2 \cdot \sin(\varphi_2) \cdot \text{atan}\left(\frac{\tan(\alpha)}{\sin(\varphi_2)}\right) \quad (6)$$

$$A = R_2^2 \cdot \sin(\varphi_1) \cdot \text{atan}\left(\frac{\sin(\varphi_1)}{\tan(\alpha)}\right) - R_1^2 \cdot \sin(\varphi_2) \cdot \text{atan}\left(\frac{\tan(\alpha)}{\sin(\varphi_2)}\right) \quad (7)$$

where α is the angle resulting from the axis defined by the intersection points of e_1 and e_3, respectively, and e_2 and e_4.

The value of α is

$$\alpha = \text{atan}\left(\frac{\tan(\varphi_2)}{\tan(\varphi_1)}\right) \quad (8)$$

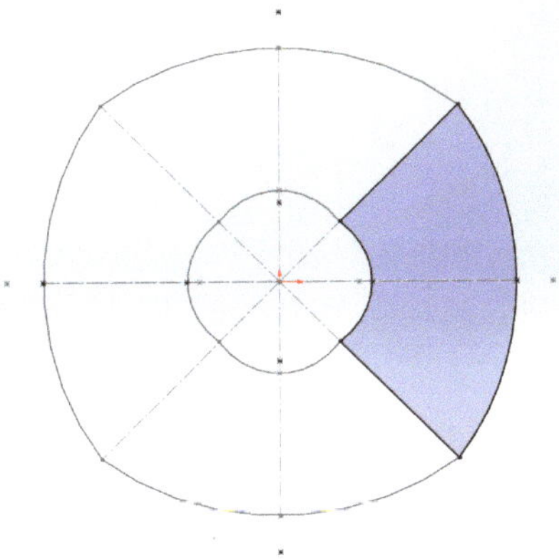

Figure 7. Representation of reachable workspace area.

Therefore, the formula for the area of the cross section of the reachable workspace is as follows:

$$A = R_2^2 \cdot \sin(\varphi_1) \cdot \text{atan}\left(\frac{\sin(\varphi_1) \cdot \tan(\varphi_1)}{\tan(\varphi_2)}\right) - R_1^2 \cdot \sin(\varphi_2) \cdot \text{atan}\left(\frac{\tan(\varphi_2)}{\sin(\varphi_2) \cdot \tan(\varphi_1)}\right) \quad (9)$$

For the determination of the volume of the reachable workspace for the 6DOF PKM, the integration of the cross-section area among the OX axis was used, taking into consideration the bounding planes defined by the first and last PR(RPR)RS kinematic chains. The geometry of the reachable workspace volume is two-fold symmetric, meaning that the whole workspace volume can be split into quarters, which aids the demonstration.

By evaluating only the quarter of the reachable workspace volume, as shown in Figure 8, by integration among the OX axis, the remaining area of the cross section in the regions bounded by the planes defined by the first and last PR(RPR)RS kinematic chains needs to be expressed in terms of the stroke among the OX axes.

Given the behavior of the sectioning plane, the following relations represent the variable area in terms of stroke among the OX axis:

$$\beta = \text{atan}\left(\frac{\sin(\varphi_1) \cdot \sqrt{R_1^2 - (x \cdot \tan(\varphi_1))^2}}{x \cdot \tan(\varphi_1)}\right) \quad (10)$$

where

$$A_2(x) = \frac{(x \cdot \tan(\varphi_1))^2 \cdot \tan(\alpha) - R_1^2 \cdot \sin(\varphi_2) \cdot \text{atan}\left(\frac{\tan(\varphi_2)}{\sin(\varphi_2) \cdot \tan(\varphi_1)}\right)}{2} \quad (11)$$

$$A_3(x) = \frac{(x \cdot \tan(\varphi_1))^2 \cdot \tan(\gamma) - R_2^2 \cdot \sin(\varphi_1) \cdot \left(\text{a}\tan\left(\frac{\sin(\varphi_1)}{\tan(\gamma)}\right) - \text{a}\tan\left(\frac{\sin(\varphi_1)}{\tan(\alpha)}\right)\right)}{2} \quad (12)$$

where

$$\gamma = \text{atan}\left(\frac{\sqrt{R_1^2 - (x \cdot \tan(\varphi_1))^2}}{x \cdot \tan(\varphi_1) \cdot \sin(\varphi_1)}\right) \quad (13)$$

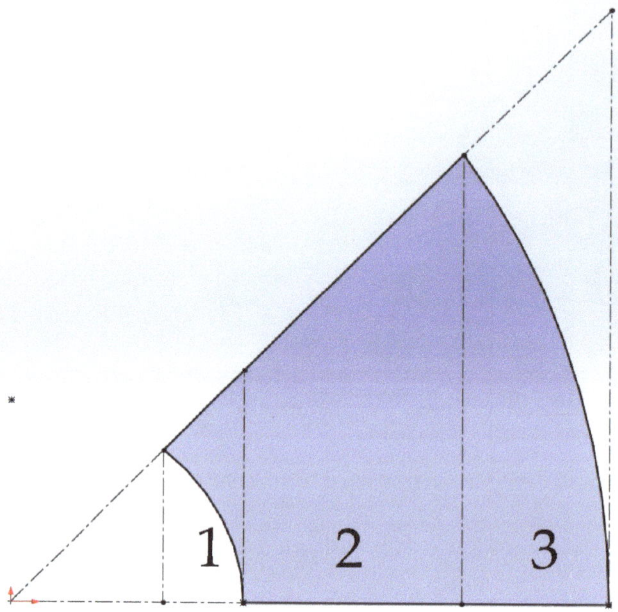

Figure 8. Representation of the half cross section ant the integration sectors.

The volume of the reachable workspace is as follows:

$$V = 4 \cdot \left(\int_{\frac{y_0}{\tan(\varphi_1)}}^{\frac{R_1}{\tan(\varphi_1)}} A_1(x)dx + \int_{\frac{R_1}{\tan(\varphi_1)}}^{\frac{y_1}{\tan(\varphi_1)}} A_2(x)dx + \int_{\frac{y_1}{\tan(\varphi_1)}}^{\frac{R_2 \cdot \sin(\varphi_1)}{\tan(\varphi_1)}} A_3(x)dx + A \cdot \frac{d}{4} \right) \tag{14}$$

where

$$y_0 = R_1 \cdot \sin(\varphi_1) \sqrt{\frac{1 - \sin(\varphi_2)^2}{1 - \sin(\varphi_1)^2 \cdot \sin(\varphi_2)^2}} \tag{15}$$

$$y_1 = R_2 \cdot \sin(\varphi_1) \sqrt{\frac{1 - \sin(\varphi_2)^2}{1 - \sin(\varphi_1)^2 \cdot \sin(\varphi_2)^2}} \tag{16}$$

3.2. Results of the Numerical Analysis

The main goal of this paper is to compare CAD optimization features for the generation of the reachable workspace of the 6DOF PKM and this requires the determination of the behavior of the volume, with respect to the tilt angles φ_1 and φ_2, as shown in Figure 9. Due to the complexity of the previous equations, explicit differentiation is not an option and the previous relations for the volume of the reachable workspace were implemented in MathWorks MATLAB and the variation in the volume was analyzed, with respect to the tilt angles, by using numerical methods.

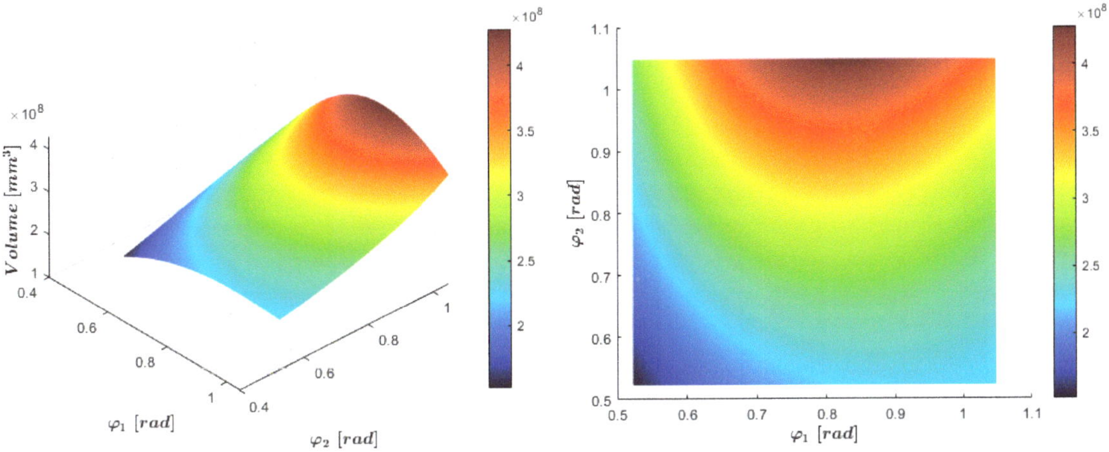

Figure 9. Representation of the volume distribution based on the values of tilt angles φ_1 and φ_2.

It was observed that the volume tends to be at its maximum around $\varphi_1 = 47.15°$ and φ_2 is the maximal value of the interval of the analysis, which, in this case, is 60°. If the analysis interval is extended up to 90°, the optimal value for φ_2 will be 90°, considering the behavior of the second P̲R(RP̲R)RS kinematic chain.

4. Implementation Based on CAD Optimization Tools

As presented in the previous sections, the PKM structure was designed and created in Catia V5 using design tools from the part, assembly and DMU Kinematics modules. The simulation process was also accomplished with the help of the CAD software Catia V5, because of the multiple algorithms offered in the module of product engineering optimizer.

In the optimizer module, we selected the following parameters with the aim of maximizing the workspace volume. The optimization parameter was determined with the smart volume function, which needs a single attribute of the modelled volume. The free parameters were as follows: the inf. range equal to 30°, the sup. range equal to 60° and the incrementation value was set to 1 degree for a more optimal result. The maximum number of updates was set to 450 and a safety parameter for the maximum number of updates was set to be equal to 50. The optimization was performed on a computer with the following hardware characteristics: CPU 3.30 GHz, memory 16 gigabytes [17].

The optimization was based on the simulated annealing algorithm as it is very stable and offers accurate results even in complex problems, as presented in the work of multiple researchers with a raw form or even a derived version [21]. The working principle is similar with the one used in metallurgy; more precisely, the process involves increasing the main parameter to the highest limit, then slowly decreasing it until it reaches the initial value [22–27]. The main parameter used for the optimization was the inclination φ_1, which is known to be equal to φ_3. Based on the selected algorithm, it was possible to obtain an extensive range, of which the most important values are presented in Table 2.

The main results summarized in Table 2 are extracted in ascending order of angle value φ_1 to expose the maximum and minimum volume limits as a relation with the tilt angle. The simulation for the PKM structure starts from the initial value of 30° and almost immediately reaches the upper limit of 60°, which follows a period of descent, until it stabilizes by itself [22–27]. The results have been post-processed to present them as clearly as possible and to draw attention to the maximum value obtained for the workspace volume. As is shown in Figure 10, the volume obtained through the module of product engineering optimizer had the maximum value of 427,839,567 mm^3, when the tilt angle φ_1 reached the value of 47.1531 deg.

Table 2. Workspace volume (mm^3) results from product engineering optimizer module (CATIA V5).

No.	Workspace Volume (mm^3)	φ_1 (deg)
1	385,427,706	30
2	388,184,667	30.4437
3	390,941,629	31.3132
4	393,698,591	33.0176
5	396,455,552	33.5412
6	399,212,514	34.5126
7	401,969,475	35.4840
8	404,726,437	36.4554
9	407,483,399	38.9554
10	410,240,360	39.8426
11	412,997,322	41.2579
12	415,754,283	42.6731
13	418,511,245	44.0884
14	421,268,207	45.5037
15	423,898,229	46.6783
16	427,839,567	47.1531
17	426,356,572	48.5324
18	425,435,343	49.6785
19	423,847,965	50.8246
20	422,363,113	51.9707
21	420,879,787	53.1168
22	419,393,133	54.2629
23	417,917,852	55.4090
24	416,427,754	56.5551
25	414,944,892	57.7012

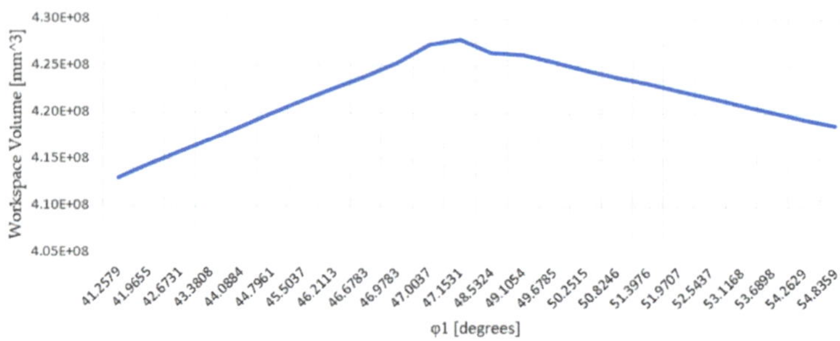

Figure 10. Graphical representation of the workspace volume optimization results from CATIA V5.

5. Conclusions

This paper presents the study that was developed to identify the working volume and its behavior based on the construction parameters of a 6-DOF parallel kinematic machine, using an analytic method and CAD optimization tools. In the article, the relations between the robot workspace and the design parameters were demonstrated, a method that can also be applied for other parallel structures. The method is useful for robot designers in the optimization of parallel robots with regard to the workspace by using CAD tools. Previous research in the field refers to the usage of CAD tools only for visual representation and not for optimizing the workspace, while this study and test results show that CAD tools are suitable for analyzing and optimizing the robot workspace of the 6DOF parallel robot, due to its easiness in application and fast time implementation time.

The result obtained from the comparison of the analytic method and the CAD optimization method showed identical behavior and almost identical results; however, due to the complexity of the analytic mathematical expressions and the way in which CatiaV5 computes volumes of bodies with complex surfaces, the optimal values obtained are approximates. The most significant results showed that there is a discrepancy between the importance of construction parameters in the case of overall reachable volume and kinematic constraints. It was determined that in order to maximize the working volume, one of the construction parameters tends to reach values at which the kinematic structure will lose degrees of freedom. Further research is proposed regarding this aspect to improve the optimization processes for the determination of the optimal working volume regarding kinematic constrains and performance indices for the PKM 6DOF structure.

Author Contributions: Conceptualization, S.-D.S. and A.O.; methodology, S.-D.S., F.P. and A.O.; software, A.O. and P.C.; validation, A.O.; formal analysis, S.-D.S. and F.P.; investigation, P.C.; resources, A.O.; data curation, A.O.; writing—original draft preparation, F.P., A.O. and P.C.; writing—review and editing, S.-D.S., F.P., A.O. and P.C.; visualization, A.O.; supervision, S.-D.S. and F.P. All authors have read and agreed to the published version of the manuscript.

Funding: This research received no external funding.

Institutional Review Board Statement: Not applicable.

Informed Consent Statement: Not applicable.

Data Availability Statement: Not applicable.

Conflicts of Interest: The authors declare no conflict of interest.

References

1. Mourtzis, D. Simulation in the design and operation of manufacturing systems: State of the art and new trends. *Int. J. Prod. Res.* **2019**, *58*, 1927–1949. [CrossRef]
2. Palpacelli, M.C.; Carbonari, L.; Palmieri, G.; D'Anca, F.; Landini, E.; Giorgi, G. Functional Design of a 6-DOF Platform for Micro-Positioning. *Robotics* **2020**, *9*, 99. [CrossRef]
3. Ahn, C.; Seo, T.; Kim, J.; Kim, T.-W. High-tilt parallel positioning mechanism development and cutter path simulation for laser micro-machining. *Comput. Aided Des.* **2007**, *39*, 218–228. [CrossRef]
4. Shimizu, Y.; Peng, Y.; Kaneko, J.; Azuma, T.; Ito, S.; Gao, W.; Lu, T.-F. Design and construction of the motion mechanism of an XY micro-stage for precision positioning. *Sens. Actuators A Phys.* **2013**, *201*, 395–406. [CrossRef]
5. Zhang, D.; Li, X.; Ni, M.; Li, P.; Dong, L.; Rui, D.; Zhang, J. Design of 6 degree-of-freedom micro-positioning mechanism for optical elements. In Proceedings of the IEEE 13th International Conference on Electronic Measurement & Instruments (ICEMI), Yangzhou, China, 20–22 October 2017.
6. Han, H.; Zhang, Y.; Zhang, H.; Han, C.; Li, A.; Xu, Z. Kinematic Analysis and Performance Test of a 6-DOF Parallel Platform with Dense Ball Shafting as a Revolute Joint. *Appl. Sci.* **2021**, *11*, 6268. [CrossRef]
7. Zhang, D.; Lang, S.Y.T. Stiffness modeling for a class of reconfigurable PKMs with three to five degrees of freedom. *J. Manuf. Syst.* **2004**, *23*, 316–327. [CrossRef]
8. Yang, J.; Xu, Z.; Wu, Q.; Zhu, M.; He, S.; Qin, C. Dynamic modeling and control of a 6-DOF micro-vibration simulator. *Mech. Mach. Theory* **2016**, *104*, 350–369. [CrossRef]
9. Shiga, Y.; Tanaka, Y.; Goto, H.; Takeda, H. Design of a six degree-of-freedom tripod parallel mechanism for flight simulators. *Int. J. Autom. Technol.* **2011**, *5*, 715–721. [CrossRef]
10. Chaudhury, A.; Ghosal, A. Determination of Workspace Volume of Parallel Manipulators Using Monte Carlo Method. In *Computational Kinematics*; Springer: Cham, Switzerland, 2018. [CrossRef]
11. Gokul, S.N.; Shrivatsan, R.; Venkatasubramanian, K.; Anjan, K.D. Deter-mination of Constant Orientation Workspace of a Stewart Platform by Geometrical Method. *Appl. Mech. Mater.* **2015**, *813–814*, 997–1001. [CrossRef]
12. Busetti, F. Simulated Annealing Overview. ResearchGate. 2001. Available online: https://www.researchgate.net/publication/238690391_Simulated_annealing_overview (accessed on 10 September 2022).
13. Leblond, T.; Froment, P.; Nazelle, P.; Sellakh, R.; Serré, P.; Chevallier, G. Gradient-based Optimization of Parameterized CAD Geometries. In Proceedings of the 11th World Congress on Structural and Multidisciplinary Optimization, Sydney, Australia, 7–12 June 2015.
14. Lucidi, S.; Sciandrone, M. A Derivative-Free Algorithm for Bound Constrained Optimization. *Comput. Optim. Appl. Kluwer Acad. Publ.* **2002**, *21*, 119–142. [CrossRef]
15. Barbarosie, C.; Lopes, S.; Toader, A.M. A gradient-type algorithm for constrained optimization with applications to multi-objective optimization of auxetic materials. *arXiv* **2018**, arXiv:1711.04863.

16. Arrouk, K.A.; Bouzgarrou, B.C.; Gogu, G. CAD based techniques for workspace analysis and representation of the 3CRS parallel manipulator. In Proceedings of the 19th International Workshop on Robotics in Alpe-Adria-Danube Region, Budapest, Hungary, 24–26 June 2010.
17. Liu, L.; Huo, J. Apple Image Segmentation Model Based on R Component with Swarm Intelligence Optimization Algorithm. *Int. J. Perform. Eng.* **2018**, *14*, 1149–1160. [CrossRef]
18. Liu, L.; Huo, J. Apple Image Recognition Multi-Objective Method Based on the Adaptive Harmony Search Algorithm with Simulation and Creation. *Information* **2018**, *9*, 180. [CrossRef]
19. Liu, L.; Huo, J.; Xue, F.; Dai, Y. Harmony Search Method with Global Sharing Factor Based on Natural Number Coding for Vehicle Routing Problem. *Information* **2020**, *11*, 86. [CrossRef]
20. Arrouk, K.A.; Bouzgarrou, B.C.; Stan, S.D.; Gogu, G. CAD Based Design Optimization of Planar Parallel Manipulators. In *Solid State Phenomena*; Trans Tech Publications, Ltd.: Bach, Switzerland, 2010. [CrossRef]
21. Stan, S.-D.; Maties, V.; Balan, R. Workspace Optimal Design of a 2 DOF Micro Parallel Robot Using Genetic Algorithms and Simulated Annealing Optimization Methods. In Proceedings of the 2007 International Conference on Mechatronics and Automation, Harbin, China, 5–8 August 2007; pp. 1108–1113. [CrossRef]
22. Popișter, F.; Oarcea, A.; Stan, S.D.; Trifan, C.V. Workspace Analysis of a Novel Parallel Kinematic Machine with 6 Degrees of Freedom. In *Advances in Manufacturing III. Manufacturing 2022. Lecture Notes in Mechanical Engineering*; Gapiński, B., Ciszak, O., Ivanov, V., Eds.; Springer: Cham, Switzerland, 2022. [CrossRef]
23. Oarcea, A.; Popister, F.; Stan, S.-D.; Cobilean, V. Comparative study of CAD optimization features for the workspace of 3DOF Parallel Robot. In Proceedings of the 2021 9th International Conference on Modern Power Systems (MPS), Cluj-Napoca, Romania, 16–17 June 2021; pp. 1–6. [CrossRef]
24. Heragu, S.S. Experimental-analysis of simulated annealing-based algorithms for the layout problem. *Eur. J. Oper. Res.* **1992**, *57*, 190–202. [CrossRef]
25. Fabian, V. Simulated annealing simulated. *Comput. Math. Appl.* **1997**, *33*, 81–94. [CrossRef]
26. Musharavati, F.; Hamouda, A.S.M. Enhanced simulated-annealing-based algorithms and their applications to process planning in reconfigurable manufacturing systems. *Adv. Eng. Softw.* **2012**, *45*, 80–90. [CrossRef]
27. Aboulissane, B.; El Haiek, D.; El Bakkali, L.; El Bahaoui, J. On The Workspace Optimization of Parallel Robots Based on CAD Approach. *Procedia Manuf.* **2019**, *32*, 1085–1092, ISSN 23519789. [CrossRef]

applied sciences

MDPI

Article

Simulation, Analysis, and Experimentation of the Compliant Finger as a Part of Hand-Compliant Mechanism Development

Dušan Stojiljković [1,*], Maša Milošević [1], Danijela Ristić-Durrant [2], Vlastimir Nikolić [1], Nenad T. Pavlović [1], Ivan Ćirić [1] and Nikola Ivačko [1]

1 Faculty of Mechanical Engineering, University of Niš, 18000 Niš, Serbia
2 Institute of Automation, University of Bremen, 28359 Bremen, Germany
* Correspondence: dusan.stojiljkovic@masfak.ni.ac.rs; Tel.: +381-642134445

Featured Application: robotics, exoskeleton development, rehabilitation robotics, grasping mechanism.

Abstract: Compliant mechanisms are gaining popularity in many different fields, such as in microelectromechanical systems (MEMS), medical applications and health care, opto-mechatronic technology, aerospace engineering, and semiconductor equipment. One of the areas for utilizing compliant mechanisms is building models of human hand counterparts. These models are often used as grasping and rehabilitation devices. Because of their properties, creating a human hand counterpart with compliant mechanisms is a much better choice compared with the models with traditional mechanisms; it looks more realistic, and its movements are much more natural compared with models with a traditional mechanism. A method of modeling and designing such a bio-inspired mechanism, as well as its experimental analysis with various forces applied, is presented in this paper. Two prototypes of the compliant fingers were obtained by 3D printing, and the calculation of the bending angle values was achieved by applying image processing to camera images of the compliant fingers' prototypes. Image processing was conducted on images taken for both loaded and unloaded 3D-printed compliant finger prototype positions. Finally, these bending angle results are compared with the results obtained by Finite Element Method (FEM) analysis and experimental results acquired by a digital protractor.

Keywords: compliant mechanism; flexure hinge; computer vision; FEM; hand rehabilitation

1. Introduction

Mechanisms produced by conventional methods do not fully resemble what nature can create. Classic hinge mechanisms are an example of this, but nevertheless, they are used in all areas of engineering due to their simplicity of operation, robustness, understanding of the operation principles, and quick and easy designing. In order to be able to create a more realistic model of the human hand, one should turn to some unconventional types of mechanisms. This can be achieved with the use of ever-increasing compliant mechanisms. In this paper, this type of mechanism is used to simulate the movement of the human hand. Such simulation can be used for many purposes, one of which is in the development of 3D model of a human hand that could be used in various applications, such as hand rehabilitation.

In order to make a hand-compliant mechanism as realistic as possible, in this paper, Finite Element Analysis (FEA) of the designed model of a human finger was first applied, followed by an experiment with the use of a digital protractor and a camera to test the position accuracy within the motion range in real conditions.

To date, published papers addressing the building of human hand mechanisms have different approaches. Observing only those that utilize the material flexibility for movement, one can classify them into two groups: those that have finger or finger-pad compliance group and those that have joint compliance. The first group uses the soft robotic approach, and the papers [1–5] show the state of the art, development, and future progress of this group. A soft touch approach is applied in this case, where the entire length of flexible elements is used for different applications. Applications of such soft gripping devices are different, such as actuators, sensors, medical tools, and rehabilitation devices. Grippers are perhaps the most abundant in this area. The study in paper [6] presents a robotic end-effector that perfectly replicates the actions of the human hand in terms of gripping and manipulating items. The soft robotic gripper shown in the paper [7] consists of three soft finger bends and one passively adaptive palm. In practice, the soft gripper could achieve a gripping force of 40 N at low actuation pressure below 100 kPa and, thus, can pick up objects of all sizes with a convex shape. Similarly, paper [8] shows a three-breasted gripper with a matched spine of each finger made of 3D-printed polylactic acid (PLA) materials sandwiched between thin-layer materials. Here, one can cite works [9] and [10], where the modeled grippers do not take the shell of the hand as a model but are free-form structures obtained by topological optimization.

A diverse series of alternative uses of structural compliance to develop simple, adaptive, compliant, and/or underactuated robotic graspers and arms that can efficiently and robustly perform various grasping and dexterous hand manipulation tasks are presented in [11].

The same study demonstrates the application based on the joints' flexibility. They represent the second group of flexible structures that use the methodology of compliant mechanisms. For the most part, these were inspired by endoskeletons used for grasping applications, and due to their external appearance, they resemble human fingers [12]. In papers [13–15], mechanisms developed in this way for the needs of the end-effector of the robotic arm are presented. The paper [16] that uses elastic ligaments and antagonistic tendons to construct anthropomorphic joints with multidirectional passive compliance as a substitute for human finger joints can be mentioned here.

Papers [17–19] show a combination of both groups, finger compliances and joint compliances, which is a new approach to soft grippers. Cited paper [18] deserves special attention. In this paper, a pressure sensor is placed on the fingertip of the elastic structure to form a soft robotic functional system. This single-build process with the advantages of multiple bodies, silicone rubber, and highly stretchable hydrogel is a popular choice for 3D printing of soft materials, which is an advantage of this approach.

Papers [20–22] show some of the ideas of how the flexibility of elements can be used in terms of hand rehabilitation. It can be said that they represent exoskeletons or endoskeletons that can be used to help people lift heavy loads and help with movement in case of immobility.

In this paper, an extension of the research that we presented in the paper [23] concerning the 3D-printed soft touch robotic manipulator is presented. In paper [23], the compliant gripper was developed as a controlled robotic manipulator to achieve smooth gripping of delicate objects where computer vision was used to collect feedback from which intelligent algorithms can control motion and grasping, and in this way, enable the gripper's ability to manipulate objects with extreme precision. The compliant gripper was created as a test to demonstrate that the presented building method enables adaptive soft touch grasping capabilities. Hence, only a limited range of gripper fingers bending angles was examined, and the gripper's design was only cursorily developed. For the purposes of extension to different applications, such as the field of hand rehabilitation, the griping compliant mechanism can be adapted to the idea of the human hand as an apparatus for some subsequent use. This adaptation is the core of the work presented in this paper in the following sections. In contrast to the paper [23], simulation, analysis, and experimentation in the range of large deformations of two compliant mechanisms obtained by the synthesis of compliant mechanisms (fabricating compliant copies of classical mechanisms, i.e., the mechanism of the human finger) were performed.

On the basis of the reviewed literature and the ever-increasing use of compliant mechanisms, this paper addresses the designed model of the human finger compliant mechanism. The paper aims to analyze the position accuracy within the motion range of this compliant finger model via FEA as well as to compare results with real-life experiments. Hence, an experimental setup with a digital camera and integrated computer vision system, which examines the position accuracy within the motion range of the loaded 3D-printed compliant finger prototypes, is presented. The paper is organized into seven sections, where in addition to the introduction given in Section 1, the design methodology with a description of the human hand, flexure hinges, and their types, and the final model of the compliant finger are described in Section 2. FEA and experiment setup are presented in Sections 3 and 4, respectively. The image processing method is presented in Section 5, and the results are in Section 6. The conclusion, overview of the results, and further research directions are given in Section 7.

2. Design Methodology

2.1. Human Hand

The human hand represents one of the most complex groups of joints and bones in the human body (together with the hand joint, it contains a sum of 54 bones out of the total 206 in the average human body). Due to its complexity, in this paper, the focus will be only on the bones and joints of the phalanges area of the human hand.

Figure 1 shows what an average human hand looks like, with all the parts that compose it. Looking at the theoretical range of motion (ROM) of hand joints, the Metacarpophalangeal (MP) and Proximal interphalangeal (PIP) joints have the largest range of motion, with a total of 135 degrees (90 degrees for flexion and -45 degrees for extension) for the MP and 100 degrees (100 degrees for flexion and 0 degrees for extension) for the PIP joint [24].

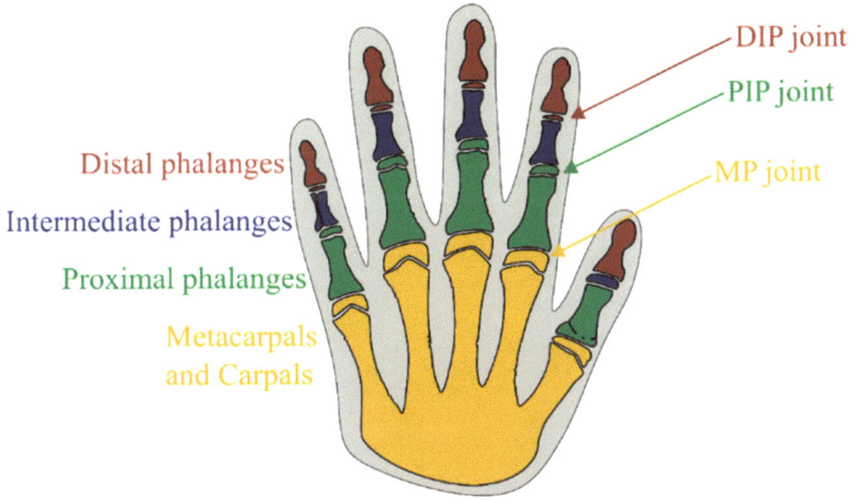

Figure 1. Anatomy of the human hand.

Hence, because of the largest flexure range, the PIP joint represents a perfect example of a joint for the analysis in this paper. The idea behind this is to achieve the bending range of the PIP joint by replacing it with a flexure hinge. All joints in the human hand can be designed this way.

2.2. Flexure Hinges

Compliant joints, otherwise called flexure hinges, are an alternative to classic, conventional joints. They allow the movement of interconnected rigid segments without the need for lubrication, noise, oscillations, and wear caused by clearance in the joints. Since they eliminate almost all the disadvantages of classic joints, they represent an ideal solution for the applications that are the core of the work presented here.

Flexure Hinge Type Selection

When deciding which type of flexure hinges to use, the application of the hinge is the most important decision criterion. In addition, the question that arises is whether the deformations are in the field of small rotations of interconnected rigid members that form a rotating pair with the joint or whether they are large deformations [25]. For these purposes, the fundamental division of flexure hinges is given in Figure 2. Notch flexure hinges (Figure 2a) and leaf springs joints (Figure 2b) are represented, as well as rod-shaped joints (Figure 2c), whose length is relatively large compared with their thickness.

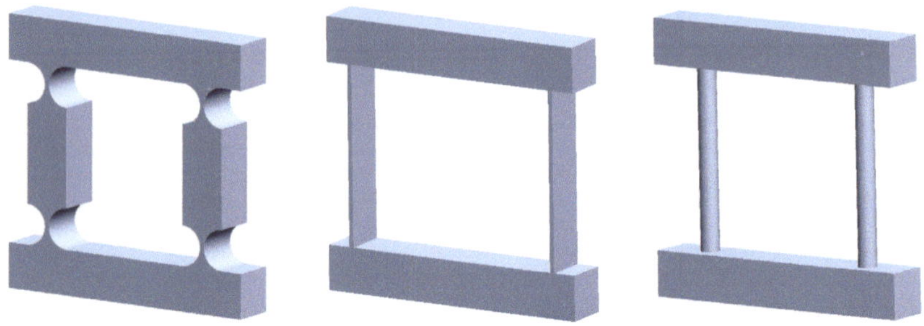

(a) (b) (c)

Figure 2. Types of compliant mechanisms with basic flexure hinges: (**a**) notch flexure hinges, (**b**) leaf springs joints, and (**c**) rod-shaped joints.

While flexure hinges in the form of leaf springs and joints in the form of rods are almost unambiguously defined, the variety of flexure hinges in the form of a notch (notch flexure hinges) is significant. Figure 3 presents a new type of notch shape for compliant joints called curved flexure hinges. For the intended application in this paper, the curved form of the notch is a perfect replacement for the joints in the human hand because they give a naturally curved position of the fingers, which is further discussed in the next section.

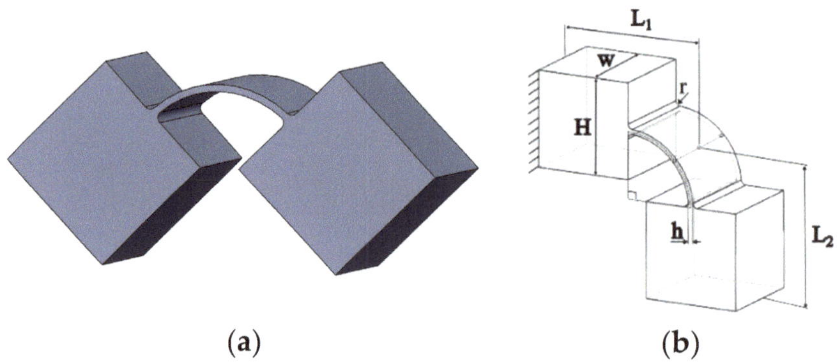

(a) (b)

Figure 3. Curved flexure hinge: (**a**) Model and (**b**) Geometrical representations.

2.3. Modeling of Compliant Finger

As already stated, the PIP joint of the index finger will be provided as a reference for modeling the flexure hinge. Figure 4 shows a human finger that will serve as an example for modeling. The lengths given in the figure represent the lengths of the finger bones together with the knuckles and, as such, will serve as limits for the given design (Figure 4a,b). In a state of relaxation (e.g., while a person is sleeping), the forearm is minimally pronated, and the wrist is kept neutral or with minor flexion and ulnar deviation. From the index through the little fingers, the MP joints are kept flexed in a gradient (45–70 degrees), while the Interphalangeal joints (IP) are in various degrees of flexion. This position is called the resting hand position [26].

In the paper [27], the resting position of the PIP joint varies from 20–47 degrees depending on the position of forearm posture and shoulder flexion. In our case, it can be noticed that the finger takes a natural resting position which, with the completely straightened position of 180 degrees, forms an angle of 21 degrees ($180^\circ - 159^\circ = 21^\circ$) (Figure 4c). This finger position was used as a reference for designing its compliant counterpart in SolidWorks version 2021 SP05.1 for modeling [28].

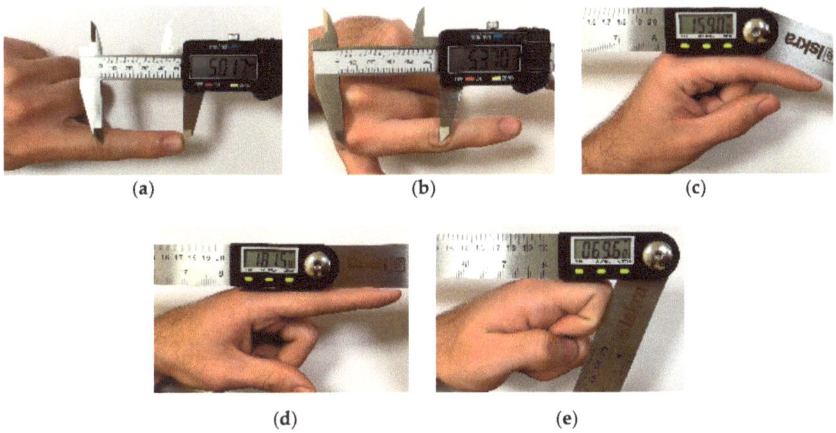

Figure 4. Measurements of the index finger: (**a**) Combined length of distal and intermediate phalanges bone and (**b**) Length of proximal phalanges bone. The angle of the PIP joint in: (**c**) A resting position, (**d**) Hyperextension, and (**e**) Flexion.

As the natural curvature of the finger was followed for modeling the compliant finger shown in Figure 4c, the PIP joint, in this case, must be modeled using a curved flexure hinge. This results in the two models shown in Figure 5 with their given dimensions of compliant fingers:

$$L_1 = 53.70 \text{ mm}$$

$$L_2 = 50.17 \text{ mm}$$

$$H = 10 \text{ mm}$$

$$w = 10 \text{ mm}$$

$$h = 1 \text{ mm}$$

$$r = 1 \text{ mm}$$

$$\alpha_1 = 21^\circ$$

$$\alpha_2 = 90^\circ$$

The first model fully follows the 21-degree bend of the finger, while the second represents an idealized model of 90-degree curved flexure hinges.

The idea is that both mechanisms will be analyzed in the following sections to determine which model is more plausible for the application considered in the paper.

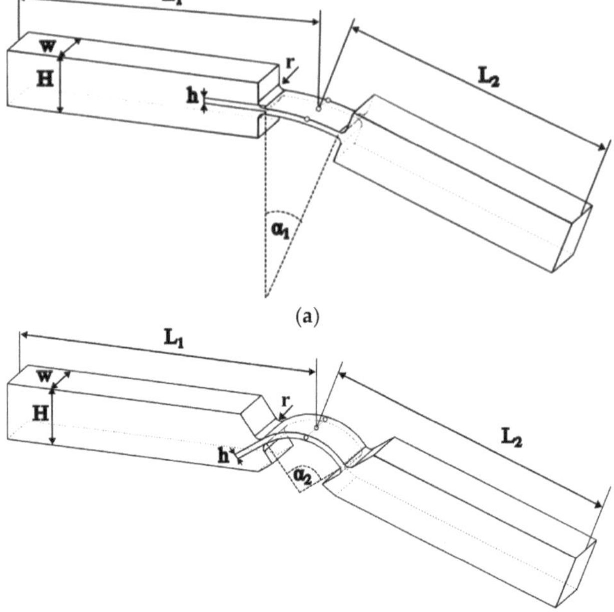

(a)

(b)

Figure 5. Compliant finger: (**a**) Curved flexure hinge with a α_1 = 21-degree bend and (**b**) Curved flexure hinge with a α_2 = 90-degree bend.

3. Finite Element Method

The Finite Element Method (FEM) was used as the basic tool for the analysis of compliant fingers [12,18]. Through the numerical solution of mathematical equations, an iterative process simulates the investigated type of mechanisms, otherwise known as Finite Element Analysis (FEA). The ANSYS software package uses this approach for the detailed analysis of the structures under investigation and was used for the analysis in this paper. Simulation and analysis were performed in ANSYS version 19.2 [29]; for them to produce valid results that can be compared with the obtained experimental results, it is necessary to fully define the given compliant mechanism. Given that compliant mechanisms dimensions are already provided as an input parameter, it is now necessary to define the material from which the compliant mechanism is constructed. For these purposes, Fused Deposition Modeling (FDM) 3D printing of Nylon material was used to create prototypes of compliant fingers. The specifications of Taulman Nylon 230 obtained from the manufacturer can be seen in Table 1 [30], and the 3D-printing process itself is described in the following.

Table 1. Mechanical properties of the 3D-printed Taulman Nylon 230.

Material Property	Taulman Nylon 230
Young's modulus, E	73 MPa
Poisson's ratio, ν	0.39
Ultimate tensile strength, σ_{max}	34 MPa
Ultimate elongation, ε_{max}	417%
Density, ρ	1.14 g/cc

Taulman Nylon 230 is a perfect option given its flexibility-to-strength ratio. With this nylon used in 3D printing, there is no snapping or brittle effect, and the parts produced are very tough, durable, and resilient. In contrast to that, the thinner sections of the 3D-printed nylon can become highly flexible. Hence, Taulman Nylon 230 is perfect for the production of compliant mechanisms prototypes and the end-use flexure components. The next step is the detailed definition of the static and dynamic characteristics given by the real conditions under which the experiment will be performed.

Figure 6 shows the defined boundary condition (fixed support A) and the load force (vector B defined in the negative direction of the horizontal axis) acting on the end of both compliant mechanisms with a 21-degree bend curved flexure hinge (Figure 6a) and a 90-degree bend curved flexure hinge (Figure 6b).

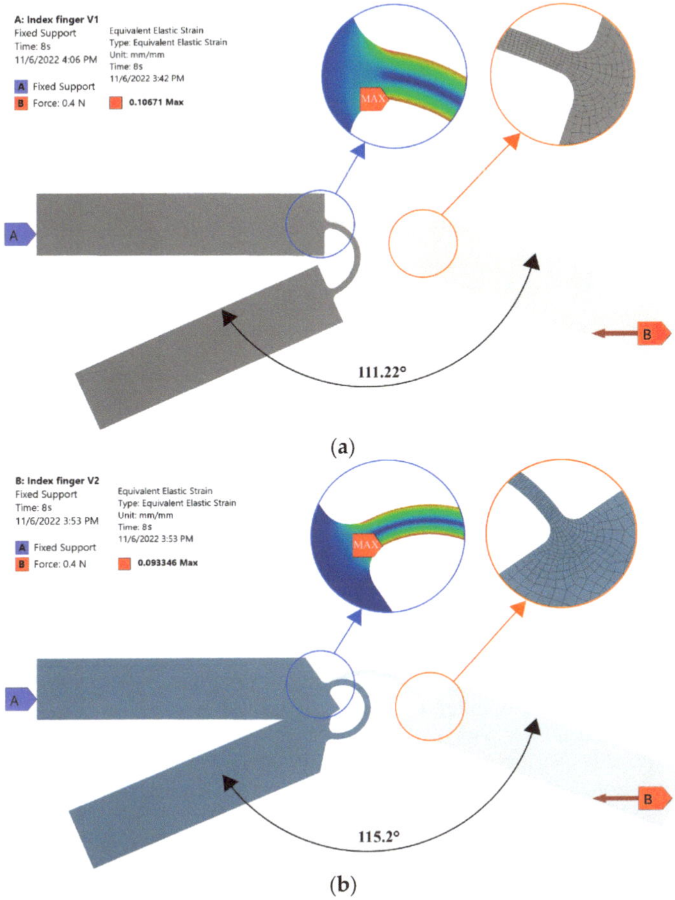

Figure 6. Boundary conditions and finite element mesh, maximal bending angle, and maximal strain of: (**a**) Curved flexure hinge with a 21-degree bend and (**b**) Curved flexure hinge with a 90-degree bend.

It is also necessary to generate a finite element mesh and its goodness is an important factor for a successful analysis. At the locations of the flexure hinges, a mesh of finite elements is produced using the "Face Meshing" function to meet the correctness of the FEA results. A complete mesh is defined with quadrilateral components of size of 0.8 mm for rigid segments of compliant mechanisms and 0.2 mm for elastic segments (flexure hinge). For a compliant mechanism with a curved flexure hinge with a 21-degree bend, the resulting mesh of the FE model contained 2298 elements and 7307 nodes, while for a compliant mechanism with a 90-degree bend, it contained 2343 elements and 7478 nodes. Non-linear FEM analysis is considered in the simulation since the static analysis takes large deflection into account. Simulation parameters maximal bending angle, and maximal strain are output parameters of interest, the results of which, in the case of maximum load force, can be seen in Figure 6.

4. Experimental Setup

For the purposes of the evaluation of the FEA results of bending angle range, measurements were performed under controlled conditions adapted to the experiment, as shown in Figure 7. For determining the bending angle of the 3D-printed finger joint, a computer vision system with Hikvision Darkfighter DS-2CD7026G0 Network IP camera was chosen. The camera was previously calibrated for the given measurement setup.

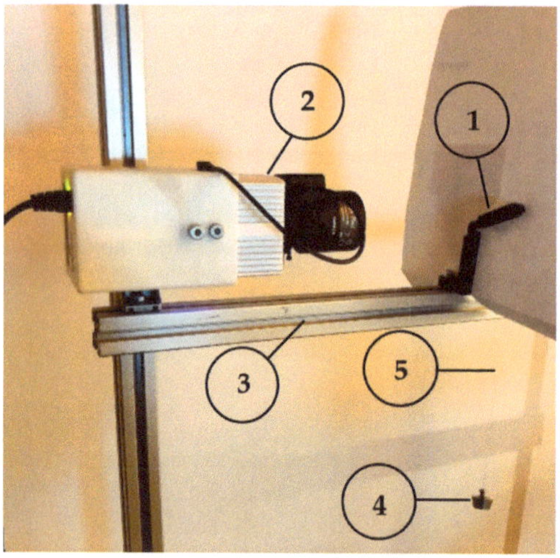

Figure 7. Experimental setup for vision-based measurement of the bending angle range of 3D-printed finger. (1) 3D-printed finger. (2) Camera. (3) Supporting structure. (4) Load. (5) Thin nonelastic string.

Figure 7 explains the experimental setup in detail, where a 3D-printed finger (1) is attached to the supporting structure (3) in the MP joint at one end, while the other end remains free. At the top of the finger, there is an opening where a thin nonelastic string (5) is pulled through and a load is connected to a string's free end (4) so that the load is perpendicular to the supporting structure. This way, the experimental setup mimics the FEA simulation. The camera (2) is placed sideways so that it captures optimal frontal projection.

For designing the technological process of 3D printing with the purpose of experimental prototypes of the compliant fingers, it is necessary to choose adequate printing parameters. The prototypes of the finger were 3D-printed on Creality Ender 5 PRO using FDM, which is a frequently applied additive manufacturing technology.

The process of creating 3D objects using filament, Taulman Nylon 230 in this case, is performed by heating the 0.4 mm diameter nozzle of the 3D printer to 235 °C, which results in the filament changing to a semi-liquid state. Layer height is 0.15 mm and is applied in each iteration, and layer by layer of material is joined with previously applied layers. All the printing parameters are listed in Table 2.

Once the prototypes were printed and the experiment setup was installed, the measurements of the motion range were taken. By recording the image of the 3D-printed prototype in different positions, it was possible to determine the path and angle of the prototype's end that occur when the load was added in the mentioned way. Processing of the recorded images was performed using a program written in Python, using the OpenCV library of algorithms.

Table 2. Parameters used for 3D-printed Taulman Nylon 230.

Printing Parameter	Value
Printing temperature	235 °C
Print bed temperature	90 °C
Bed surface	Glass
Layer height	0.15 mm
Nozzle diameter	0.4 mm
Flexure hinge infill	100%
Color	Black
Nominal diameters of the filament	1.75 mm

Weights of 10 g, 20 g, 30 g, and 40 g were added one after the other in order to determine the maximal 3D-printed compliant finger bending angle (as described in the previous section). Images were taken for each position of the measurement series when the system was in balance, and after that, the angles were measured using computer vision. The system remained unloaded between each measurement until it returned to its original position.

The results of measurements after image processing were compared with manual measurements using a digital protractor, and they are presented and discussed in the Section 6.

5. Image Processing

For the experiment, computer vision was used to approximate the bending angle of the finger joint. The use of image processing for this type of experiment setup ensures an accurate approach to collecting measurements, which means that, apart from the calculation error, the measurement error is reduced to the initial marking of the object and the appropriate placement of the camera (both calibrations are addressed in the first instance of the experiment). The advantage of setting up an experiment with a high color contrast in the imaged scene lies in the fact that black and white image regions have a distinct difference in pixel values between the object and the background, which helps in detecting the desired object region. In the presented experiment, 3D-printed finger of black color is placed on the white background. The image processing task is divided into two parts: recognizing the segment of the joint of the 3D-printed finger that bears the load and determining the bending angle when the joint is loaded.

The camera records the video from which the necessary images are extracted (in the initial position of the 3D-printed finger and under the mentioned loaded case) for real-time object detection. One of the most effective object detection techniques that serve as a point of reference for object detection in computer vision projects is the bounding-box-based object detection. Bounding-box detections are represented by outlining the rectangles, which fully bound the objects in the image, with the x- and y-image coordinates of the rectangles' centers, as well as with the width, and height of the rectangles. After that, the bending angle about the y-axis (vertical axis of the image coordinate system) is calculated. As was said in Section 4, image processing is performed using a program written in Python, using the OpenCV library of algorithms with the function cv2.MinAreaRect(). The cv2.MinAreaRect() function employs the rotating calipers approach to identify the minimal rectangle that encompasses the object region in the image. First, the original image (Figure 8 left) is segmented using thresholding-based segmentation. The rectangle extraction procedure begins by determining the convex hull of the set of points on the boundary of segmented object region and subsequently rotating a line segment, known as "calipers" around the convex hull while measuring the dimensions of the rectangle created by the calipers and convex hull during each rotation. The rectangle with the least area is selected as the minimum area rectangle.

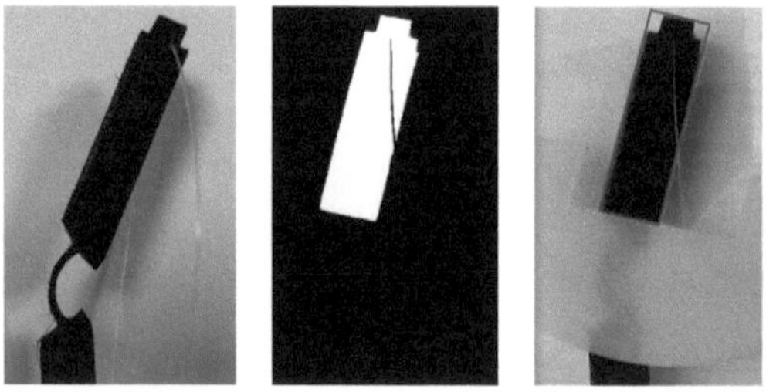

Figure 8. Object detection using image processing. (**left**) Original image of the 3D-printed finger. (**middle**) Segmented object region represented with white pixels in the segmented binary image. (**right**) Detected object bounded with an extracted minimal rectangle (blue-colored rectangle).

Figure 8 shows an example of extracting an object using the function cv2.minAreaRect() [31], which extracts a rectangle (bounding box) of the smallest area around the desired shape. The lower portion of the compliant finger that is being imaged is covered to guarantee that just the rectangle that is of interest for the presented analysis, i.e., the rectangle with the smallest area, will be extracted.

Figure 9 shows an example of a loaded finger joint using the developed function for measuring the bending angle about the y-axis (vertical axis of the image coordinate system). A segment of interest is isolated by markers of contrasting color value because the algorithm separates pixels of low and high color properties (hue, color saturation, and value) and then identifies the largest morphologically closed contour inside the processed image.

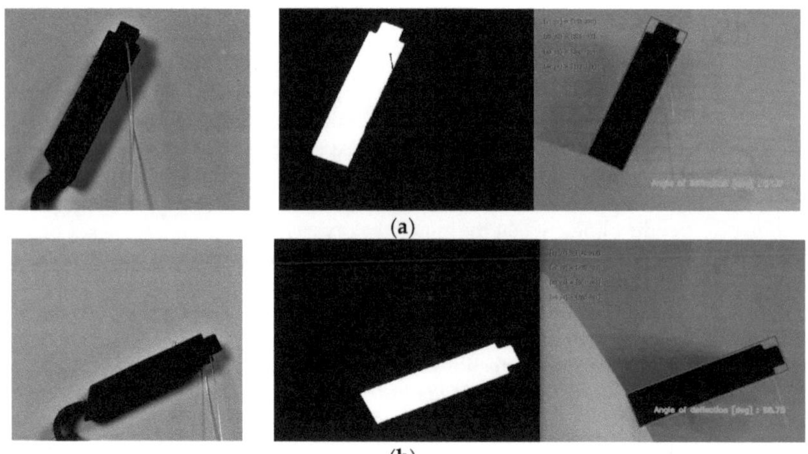

Figure 9. Example of different joint positions: (**a**) unloaded and (**b**) loaded. Original images (left column) of the 3D-printed finger. Segmented object regions represented with white pixels in the segmented binary images (middle column). Detected object bounded with an extracted minimal rectangle represented by blue-colored rectangle (right column).

The value shown in Figure 9a is the initial position, while Figure 9b represents the difference between the found bending angle and the image coordinate system y-axis.

6. Results and Discussion

Table 3 shows the results obtained by experimental measurement of the bending angle of the 3D-printed finger using computer vision, manual measurement with an electronic protractor, and numerical results obtained by FEA.

Table 3. Results for the bending angle θ measured at the endpoint of compliant finger.

Flexure Hinge Type	Method	Force (N)			
		≈0.1	**≈0.2**	**≈0.3**	**≈0.4**
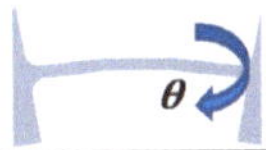	Computer Vision	31.9°	69°	94.1°	124.2°
	Protractor Measurement	32.7°	68.7°	93°	126.9°
	FEA	70.854°	110.98°	126.57°	134.96°
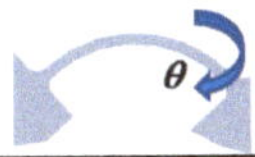	Computer Vision	34.9°	68.5°	92.8°	123.3°
	Protractor Measurement	33.5°	68.1°	92.1°	121.7°
	FEA	79.54°	115.09°	129.14°	135.93°

As can be noticed, FEA results show a large error with respect to experimentally measured values in cases where small loads were applied, while in cases of maximum loading, this error is reduced. FEA shows that both compliant fingers have very similar results in output angles but still provide better results for a curved flexure hinge with a 90-degree bend. On the other hand, the experiment shows that a 21-degree bend curved flexure hinge provides better results. The reason for that can be contained in the assumption that the information provided by the material manufacturer is different for the filament used for 3D-printed prototypes of fingers.

In order to prove this assumption, a tensile test was performed to determine the material properties of 3D-printed test specimens (Figure 10). The tensile test was performed according to the international standard ISO 527-2, which determines the tensile properties of molding and extrusion plastics. In Figure 10a, the test specimen at the beginning of the tensile test (without a load) can be seen, and in Figure 10b, the test specimen during the load stage is shown.

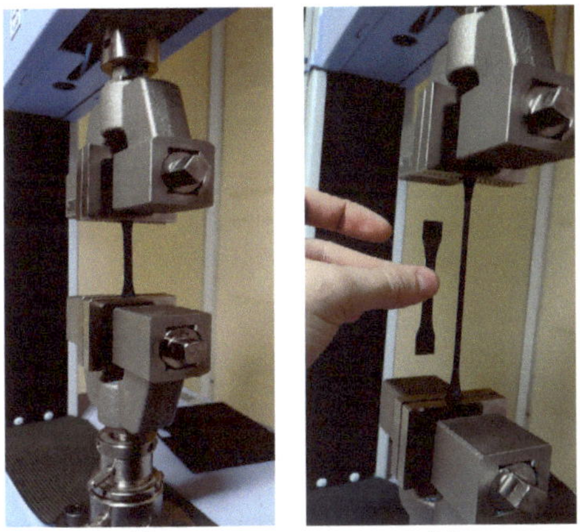

(a) (b)

Figure 10. The setup for tensile testing: (**a**) unloaded test tube and (**b**) loaded test tube.

As a result of the tensile test for the 3D-printed Taulman Nylon 230 material, the stress–strain curve shown in Figure 11 was obtained. The orange line illustrates the hypothetical straight line that the material would follow if it were constantly in the area of elasticity (in the region where Hook's law applies), whereas the blue line depicts the actual behavior of this material when it is stretched. The slope of the straight-line portion of the stress–strain curve can be utilized to define the modulus of elasticity (Young's modulus). Special attention should be paid to the instant of the stress point where the material enters the non-linear deformation region (i.e., when the blue and the orange lines diverge), as this is the region where the compliant fingers material is when the large angular deformations take place.

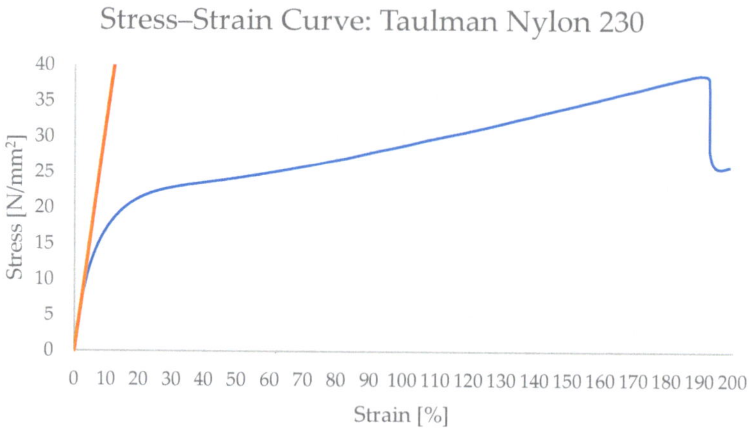

Figure 11. The stress–strain curve obtained from tensile testing data. (**blue**) True stress–strain curve. (**orange**) Hypothetical straight line of pure elastic behavior of the material.

All the values of the mechanical parameters required for the simulation and FEA are determined by examining the data collected from the performed tensile test. The entire set of mechanical parameters for the 3D-printed Taulman Nylon 230 material is presented in Table 4. As can be observed, the acquired Young's modulus is nearly 4.5 times greater than the manufacturer's Young's modulus (manufacturer's Young's modulus—73 MPa; Young's modulus obtained by tensile test—325 MPa), while ultimate tensile strength is not that different.

Table 4. Mechanical properties of the 3D-printed Taulman Nylon 230 obtained by tensile testing.

Material Property	Taulman Nylon 230
Young's modulus, E	325 MPa
Poisson's ratio, ν	0.39
Ultimate tensile strength, σ_{max}	38.8 MPa
Yield strength, σ_y	7.9 MPa

With the experimentally acquired mechanical characteristics, FEA of the compliant fingers was carried out. The FEA setup was the same as that described in Section 3, with a few additional improvements. A mesh is now defined as a size of 0.2 mm for rigid segments of compliant mechanisms and 0.05 mm for elastic segments (flexure hinge). This was implemented in order to ensure the repeatability of the FEA results, which has a stress convergence test tolerance below 1%. A compliant mechanism with a curved flexure hinge with a 21-degree bend now has the resulting mesh of the FE model, which contains 32,615 elements and 33,425 nodes, while a compliant mechanism with a 90-degree bend contained 34,552 elements and 34,552 nodes. The force with which the compliant fingers were loaded in the simulation corresponds to the product of the mass of the weights (from the initial 10 g to 60 g) with which the experiments were performed and the gravitational acceleration obtained at the site where the experiment was performed (the value of the gravitational acceleration for the city of Niš, Serbia, is 9.80408 m/s^2). Adding forces corresponding to weights of 50 and 60 g was necessary so that in FEA, we could obtain results of maximum bending angles that correspond to the theoretical range of motion for the PIP joint of 100 degrees. The resulting forces and deflection angles obtained by FEA can be seen in Figure 12. The difference between bending angles for the two types of compliant fingers can be clearly seen. Better angle results are produced by a compliant finger with a 90-degree bend curved flexure hinge (red line), which is visible even at modest load levels.

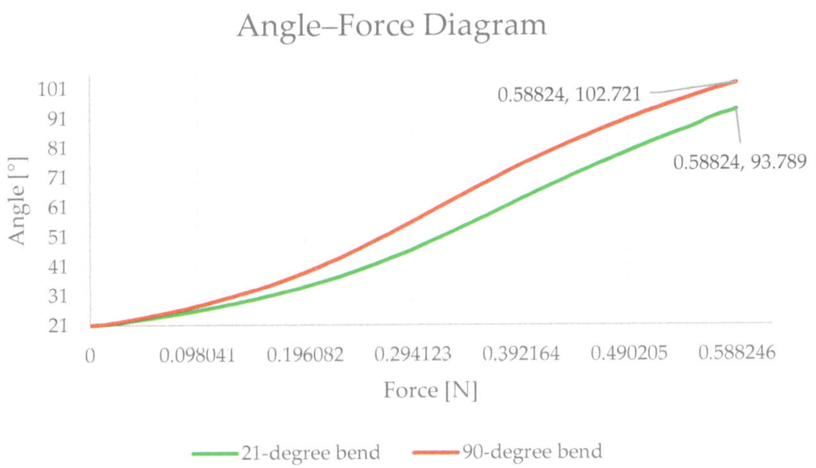

Figure 12. Angle–force diagram for compliant fingers obtained by FEA.

The above results should be seen as results in terms of internal stress and strain. In Figure 13, it can be seen that the compliant finger with a 90-degree bend curved flexure hinge has minor stress through the entire range of angular deformations. The maximal stress in the end position at the highest load force for a 90-degree bend curved flexure hinge is 17.324 MPa for bending angle θ = 102.721°, and for a 21-degree bend curved flexure hinge, it is 17.406 MPa for bending angle θ = 93.789°.

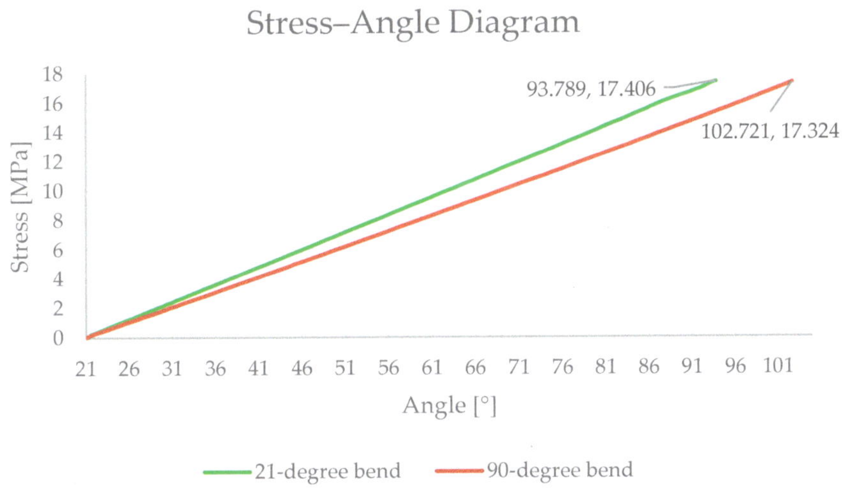

Figure 13. Stress–angle diagram for compliant fingers obtained by FEA.

As a result of all the above, it was necessary to repeat the experimental measurement in order to provide the values of the angles for the weights of 50 and 60 g so that we could perform a comparison with the FEA. Therefore, two new prototypes of compliant fingers were 3D-printed, which served us for the desired experimentation. This opportunity was used to repeat the already conducted experiment once more, ensuring the outcome results of the earlier experiment (Figure 14).

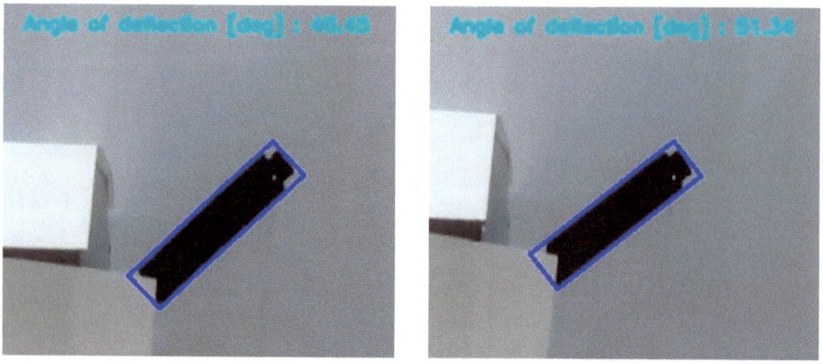

(a) **(b)**

Figure 14. Example of computer vision measured bending angle θ for compliant finger with (**a**) curved flexure hinge with a 21-degree bend and (**b**) curved flexure hinge with a 90-degree bend, for a loaded 30 g weight.

Table 5 shows the newly obtained results of the experiment (Computer Vision Method) and FEA. The results presented in this way clearly confirm the similarity between FEA and experimental results in the area up to 70 degrees for curved flexure hinge with a 21-degree bend and up to 80 degrees for curved flexure hinge with a 90-degree bend. In the area larger than the above-mentioned angles, the results diverge. This outcome can be attributed to the behavior of the material, which in the area of large deformations tends to creep after the addition of weights heavier than 40 g. With the graphic in Figure 13, this can be confirmed because, in these areas, the stress is greater than 12 MPa for both compliant fingers. This also refers to Figure 11, where, as already noted, the material enters the non-linear deformation region.

Table 5. New results for the bending angle θ measured at the endpoint of compliant fingers.

Flexure Hinge Type	**Method**	**Force (N)**					
		≈0.1	**≈0.2**	**≈0.3**	**≈0.4**	**≈0.5**	**≈0.6**
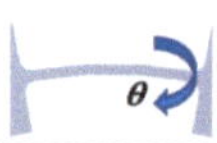	Computer Vision	26.57°	33.18°	46.45°	68.01°	99.46°	124.81°
	FEA	25.917°	34.033°	46.687°	63.393°	79.764°	93.789°
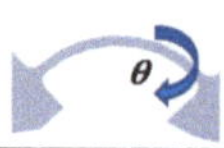	Computer Vision	26.34°	37.67°	51.34°	77.47°	108.12°	133.96°
	FEA	27.53°	38.85°	56.01°	75°	90.741°	102.72°

The difference between the previously performed experiment (Table 3) and the newly performed experiment (Table 5) should also be explained. The conclusion of the difference in results is explained by the fact that the previous experiment was performed after the bending test of 3D-printed compliant finger prototypes. This means that the prototypes were previously brought to a state of large deformations, whereby plastic deformation remained in the material. It should be noted that these permanent deformations were not seen and that the prototypes had the ability to return to their initial state, but the experiment performed with such plastic deformations in the material cannot be considered valid.

7. Conclusions

In this paper, a model of a compliant mechanism that is a counterpart to the human hand was discussed. For this purpose, compliant mechanisms are the perfect choice due to their properties and benefits compared with traditional mechanisms, such as no need for lubrication, no noise or oscillations, and wear caused by clearance in the joints. Therefore, two types of compliant fingers were analyzed. Prototypes with curved flexure hinges of mentioned fingers were 3D-printed in order to experimentally prove which of these two types represents a more adequate solution. Such models can be used in various applications, such as robotic grasping devices that simulate the movements of a human hand, interactive video gaming, and hand rehabilitation [32]. In the case of hand rehabilitation, the discussed models could be used as parts of the hand exoskeletons for patients with impaired hand fingers' movements or parts of the "movement training by imitation" rehabilitation systems, where the patient would be asked to imitate the movement of the fingers' models teleoperated by the therapist or intelligently controlled to demonstrate particular movements of the figures and hand gestures.

Presented simulations and parametric analyzes were performed to demonstrate the accuracy of the software analysis to correspond with the experimental results and, thus, to use this method for further research. The initially obtained results showed a poor correlation between experimental and FEA results. The assumption was made that the information provided by the material manufacturer was different from the filament used for 3D-printed prototypes of compliant fingers. This is a common mistake when experimenting with 3D-printed prototypes.

As a solution, adequate measurements should be taken to obtain the correct specifications for 3D-printed compliant fingers and set the correct parameters for the FEA simulation. To demonstrate this possible solution, tensile test was performed to determine the material properties of the 3D-printed test specimens, which were used for the re-executed FEA.

The newly obtained results showed a good correlation between experimental and FEA results. In the areas of low and medium deformations, the agreement of FEA and experimental results could be seen within the limits of less than 10%. The limit increases to 25% in regions with high deformations. This discrepancy can be attributed to the fact that the printed elements are often not of homogeneous structure, while the model obtained by simulation is completely idealized. It should also be emphasized that the program in which the analysis was performed does not provide optimal results related to the non-linear area of deformations.

The next step would be to implement such a method for the case of a compliant finger that would have all the necessary joints that would allow the realistic range of motion that human fingers have. The analysis of such a compliant finger would complete the entire development of the hand-compliant mechanism, which could later be used in various applications, such as the hand rehabilitation device mentioned above, with the help of adequate control for its actuation.

Author Contributions: Conceptualization, D.S., N.T.P. and I.Ć.; Methodology, D.S. and M.M.; Software, M.M. and N.I.; Validation, N.T.P.; Formal analysis, D.S.; Investigation, M.M. and N.I.; Resources, I.Ć. and N.I.; Data curation, I.Ć.; Writing—original draft, D.S. and M.M.; Writing—review & editing, D.R.-D., N.T.P. and I.Ć.; Visualization, D.S. and M.M.; Supervision, D.R.-D. and N.T.P.; Project administration, D.R.-D. and V.N.; Funding acquisition, D.R.-D., V.N., N.T.P. and I.Ć. All authors have read and agreed to the published version of the manuscript.

Funding: This research was financially supported by the Ministry of Science, Technological Development and Innovation of the Republic of Serbia (Contract No. 451-03-47/2023-01/ 200109 and partly by the Innovation Fund of the Republic of Serbia through the Innovation Voucher I.D. 1209 "Development of a Robotic End Effector for the Soft Touch Application".

Institutional Review Board Statement: Not applicable.

Informed Consent Statement: Informed consent was obtained from all subjects involved in the study.

Data Availability Statement: Not applicable.

Conflicts of Interest: The authors declare no conflict of interest.

References

1. Manti, M.; Cacucciolo, V.; Cianchetti, M. Stiffening in Soft Robotics: A Review of the State of the Art; Stiffening in Soft Robotics: A Review of the State of the Art. *IEEE Robot. Autom. Mag.* **2016**, *23*, 93–106. [CrossRef]
2. Wang, H.; Totaro, M.; Beccai, L. Toward Perceptive Soft Robots: Progress and Challenges. *Adv. Sci.* **2018**, *5*, 1800541. [CrossRef] [PubMed]
3. Walker, J.; Zidek, T.; Harbel, C.; Yoon, S.; Strickland, F.S.; Kumar, S.; Shin, M. Soft Robotics: A Review of Recent Developments of Pneumatic Soft Actuators. *Actuators* **2020**, *9*, 3. [CrossRef]
4. Gul, J.Z.; Sajid, M.; Rehman, M.M.; Siddiqui, G.U.; Shah, I.; Kim, K.-H.; Lee, J.-W.; Choi, K.H. 3D printing for soft robotics—A review. *Sci. Technol. Adv. Mater.* **2018**, *19*, 243–262. [CrossRef]
5. Polygerinos, P.; Correll, N.; Morin, S.A.; Mosadegh, B.; Onal, C.D.; Petersen, K.; Cianchetti, M.; Tolley, M.T.; Shepherd, R.F. Soft Robotics: Review of Fluid-Driven Intrinsically Soft Devices; Manufacturing, Sensing, Control, and Applications in Human-Robot Interaction. *Adv. Eng. Mater.* **2017**, *19*, 1700016. [CrossRef]
6. Deimel, R.; Brock, O. A novel type of compliant and underactuated robotic hand for dexterous grasping. *Int. J. Robot. Res.* **2016**, *35*, 161–185. [CrossRef]
7. Zhou, J.; Chen, S.; Wang, Z. A Soft-Robotic Gripper with Enhanced Object Adaptation and Grasping Reliability. *IEEE Robot. Autom. Lett.* **2017**, *2*, 2287–2293. [CrossRef]
8. Gao, Y.; Huang, X.; Mann, I.; Su, H.J. A Novel Variable Stiffness Compliant Robotic Gripper Based on Layer Jamming. *J. Mech. Robot.* **2020**, *12*, V05BT07A017. [CrossRef]
9. Liu, C.H.; Huang, G.; Chiu, C.; Pai, T.Y. Topology Synthesis and Optimal Design of an Adaptive Compliant Gripper to Maximize Output Displacement. *J. Intell. Robot. Syst. Theory Appl.* **2018**, *90*, 287–304. [CrossRef]
10. Milojević, A.; Pavlović, N.; Linß, S.; Tomić, M.; Pavlović, N.; Handroos, H. A concept of adaptive two finger gripper with embedded actuators. *Mech. Mach. Sci.* **2017**, *45*, 239–250. [CrossRef]
11. Chang, C.M.; Gerez, L.; Elangovan, N.; Zisimatos, A.; Liarokapis, M. On alternative uses of structural compliance for the development of adaptive robot grippers and hands. *Front. Neurorobot.* **2019**, *13*, 91. [CrossRef] [PubMed]
12. Tavakoli, M.; Sayuk, A.; Lourenço, J.; Neto, P. Anthropomorphic finger for grasping applications: 3D printed endoskeleton in a soft skin. *Int. J. Adv. Manuf. Technol.* **2017**, *91*, 2607–2620. [CrossRef]
13. Lotti, F.; Vassura, G. A novel approach to mechanical design of articulated fingers for robotic hands. In Proceedings of the IEEE/RSJ International Conference on Intelligent Robots and Systems, Lausanne, Switzerland, 30 September–4 October 2002; Volume 2, pp. 1687–1692. [CrossRef]
14. Lotti, F.; Tiezzi, P.; Vassura, G.; Zucchelli, A. Mechanical Structures for Robotic Hands based on the 'Compliant Mechanism' Concept. In Proceedings of the 7th ESA Workshop on Advanced Space Technologies for Robotics and Automation 'ASTRA 2002' ESTEC, Noordwijk, The Netherlands, 19–21 November 2002; pp. 1–8.
15. Kontoudis, G.P.; Liarokapis, M.; Vamvoudakis, K.; Furukawa, T. An adaptive actuation mechanism for anthropomorphic robot hands. *Front. Robot. AI* **2019**, *6*, 47. [CrossRef] [PubMed]
16. Çulha, U.; Iida, F. Enhancement of finger motion range with compliant anthropomorphic joint design. *Bioinspir. Biomim.* **2016**, *11*, 026001. [CrossRef] [PubMed]
17. Zhou, J.; Chen, X.; Li, J.; Tian, Y.; Wang, Z. A soft robotic approach to robust and dexterous grasping. In Proceedings of the 2018 IEEE International Conference on Soft Robotics (RoboSoft), Livorno, Italy, 24–28 April 2018; pp. 412–417. [CrossRef]
18. Kaur, M.; Kim, W.S. Toward a Smart Compliant Robotic Gripper Equipped with 3D-Designed Cellular Fingers. *Adv. Intell. Syst.* **2019**, *1*, 1900019. [CrossRef]
19. Zhu, W.; Lu, C.; Zheng, Q.; Fang, Z.; Che, H.; Tang, K.; Zhu, M.; Liu, S.; Wang, Z. A Soft-Rigid Hybrid Gripper with Lateral Compliance and Dexterous In-hand Manipulation. *arXiv* **2021**, arXiv:2110.10035. [CrossRef]
20. Meng, Q.; Shen, Z.; Nie, Z.; Meng, Q.; Wu, Z.; Yu, H. Modeling and Evaluation of a Novel Hybrid-Driven Compliant Hand Exoskeleton Based on Human-Machine Coupling Model. *Appl. Sci.* **2021**, *11*, 10825. [CrossRef]
21. Luhmann, O. Development of a Novel Hand Exoskeleton for the Rehabilitation and Assistance of Upper Motor Neuron Syndrome Patients. Master's Thesis, KTH Royal Institute of Technology, University of Stockholm, Stockholm, Sweden, 2020.
22. Zaid, A.M.; Chean, T.; Sukor, J.; Hanafi, D. Development of hand exoskeleton for rehabilitation of the post-stroke patient. *AIP Conf. Proc.* **2017**, *1891*, 020103. [CrossRef]
23. Ivan, Ć.; Nikola, I.; Dušan, S.; Stefan, L.; Petar, Đ.; Milan, P.; Nenad, T.P. Development and Control of 3D Printed Soft Touch Robotic Manipulator. 2022, pp. 257–260. Available online: http://www.eventiotic.com/eventiotic/library/paper/726 (accessed on 27 October 2022).
24. Ngeo, J.G.; Tamei, T.; Shibata, T. Continuous and simultaneous estimation of finger kinematics using inputs from an EMG-to-muscle activation model. *J. NeuroEng. Rehabil.* **2014**, *11*, 122. [CrossRef]
25. Pavlović, N.D.; Pavlović, N.T. *Gipki Mehanizmi*; Mašinski fakultet, Univerziteta u Nišu: Niš, Serbia, 2013. (In Serbian)
26. Sridhar, K. Functional Anatomy and Biomechanics of the Hand. In *Textbook of Plastic, Reconstructive, and Aesthetic Surgery*; Thieme Medical and Scientific Publishers: Noida, India, 2018. [CrossRef]
27. Lee, K.S.; Jung, M.C. Flexion and Extension Angles of Resting Fingers and Wrist. *Int. J. Occup. Saf. Ergon.* **2014**, *20*, 91–101. [CrossRef]
28. Available online: https://www.solidworks.com/ (accessed on 10 April 2022).

29. Available online: https://www.ansys.com/ (accessed on 23 April 2022).
30. Technical Data Sheet (TDS): Nylon 230. p. 230. Available online: https://taulman3d.com/nylon-230-spec.html (accessed on 23 April 2022).
31. Available online: https://docs.opencv.org/3.4/dd/d49/tutorial_py_contour_features.html (accessed on 23 September 2022).
32. Aggogeri, F.; Mikolajczyk, T.; O'Kane, J. Robotics for rehabilitation of hand movement in stroke survivors. *Adv. Mech. Eng.* **2019**, *11*, 1687814019841921. [CrossRef]

applied sciences

MDPI

Communication

Aspects Related to the Design and Manufacturing of an Original and Innovative Marker Support System for Use in Clinical Optometry

Victor Constantin, Daniel Besnea, Bogdan Gramescu and Edgar Moraru *

Department of Mechatronics and Precision Mechanics, Faculty of Mechanical Engineering and Mechatronics, University Politehnica of Bucharest, 060042 Bucharest, Romania
* Correspondence: edgar.moraru@upb.ro

Abstract: The compliant mechanism studied in this paper is used in the structure of an assembly necessary for the temporary mounting of visual markers on glasses frames. Proper correction of vision defects in patients is a field of study in healthcare that has grown in complexity, along with all aspects of technology, over the past decades. As such, along with better lenses and frames, including custom solutions, the devices used to determine the patient's specific parameters need to be more complex and precise. However, this is only part of the problem: while many devices exist that take measurements such as interpupillary distance with great precision, these come at a very high cost and do not take into account aspects related to real-life usage of the lenses, such as the patient's position, angle, etc. Given the considerations above, this paper approaches the design, simulation, realization and testing of a working model of a frame used to support markers used in the optometry process. The design proposed in this paper assumes that the system used can be used while the glasses are mounted on the patient's face, without influencing in any way their position in front of the patient's eyes. Furthermore, the system must allow assembly and disassembly with minimal effort, to allow the patient to perform some movements without changing the position of the frame, as well as the easy access to the markers mounted on the spectacle frame. The main scope of the paper is to design and choose the correct constructive solution of a compliant mechanism for this important clinical optometric application in terms of geometric parameters, material and technology used to obtain appropriate performances. The authors highlight how the parameters and manufacturing technology for the device were chosen, and a finite element analysis is used to simulate the mechanical behaviour of the mechanism and to choose the optimal variant in terms of the desired displacement between three proposed materials for the given application. After justifying the choice of the constructive solution, several physical models of optometric support markers were realised using Fused Deposition Modeling (FDM), and Polyethylene terephthalate glycol (PETG) or polylactic acid as materials. Furthermore, an electro-pneumatic experimental test stand was developed to simulate and test the functionality of the device and to validate the proposed model.

Keywords: compliant mechanism; optometry; 3D printing; finite element analysis

1. Introduction

The use of multiple types of measuring systems is widespread in the field of optometry, and specialists rely on such devices along with specific methods to determine a patient's specific needs in regard to customizing lenses. In this regard, certain aspects of measuring these parameters are perceived as being mandatory, such as determining the user's perceived effect of the lenses on vision in a real-world environment: reading a computer screen, a book, looking in the distance. One such aspect is that the glasses and lenses should be mounted on the patient's face, and their position should not be in any way modified by the measuring apparatus. This is especially true when it comes to personalised progressive lenses. As such, certain requirements have been identified, as explained below:

- High elasticity—the mount should allow for usage with a wide array of models of glasses.
- Maximum weight 5 g—total weight of the system will be two such mechanisms, for a total of 10 g. It was considered that the mounting bracket should not be heavier than one of the lightest pairs of glasses. This is mostly an empirical parameter, based on previous iterations of such systems.
- Good resistance to repeated usage—the system should not be prone to easily breaking while being used for multiple dimensions of seeing glasses.
- Easy to manufacture, but especially easy to modify between product iterations due to the shifting fashions in eyewear; the mounting bracket should easily follow suit.
- Low cost and good aesthetics
- Made in one part—measuring accuracy will greatly depend on how well the system is assembled. Related to this last point, a special model of a compliant mechanism that achieves the transmission of force and motion through its own elastic body transformation was proposed. Through several iterations, a shape was obtained, mostly being designed around the normal shape of a user's glasses frames.

Figure 1 shows two views of the proposed mechanism (side and isometric view), which is equipped with two handles.

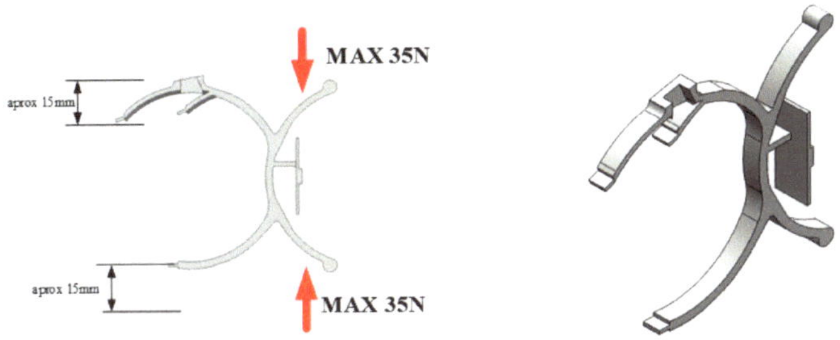

Figure 1. General view of mechanism.

A force of approximately 35 N (each) will be exerted on them, which is necessary to open the mechanism with a total stroke of 30 mm. The forces necessary to open the mechanism are determined following the study in the specialized literature [1], and of some simple tests performed in the laboratory—allowing an average user to open the device with minimal effort.

Similar systems have been developed for use in the field of optometry. Such systems, currently employed throughout optometry clinics allow for easy measurement, with relatively low errors of a small number of parameters, such as interpupillary distance, total, left and right, as well as a basic calculation of the boxing parameters needed when cutting and fitting the lens to a specific frame. One such example is the VisionFit Dispensing System [2], which allows for measurement of interpupillary distances both for near and far, boxing measurements, as well as some fitting parameters of the frames. This system does not, however, allow for complex measurements to be taken (curvature of frames and pantoscopic angle). Another such system is the Optikam [3], which allows measurement of a much larger number of parameters, but does feature a very large and complex system for attaching the markers to the patient's face, and thus runs the risk of interfering with the natural position the frame would otherwise have on the patient's face. Another such system is the DigiFit, which allows for measurements of a large number of parameters, but does, however, generally require the lens to be taken out of the frame. Since some corrections, such as squinting, are made by the lens, a complex system must be employed to allow for corrections to the lens's optic centre [4].

While the systems presented thus far allow for some parameters to be measured, there are systems under use that allow for all parameters to be obtained. These, however, are very expensive and usually require special training and occupy a large part of the clinic for use. One such system is the highly capable ZEISS i.Terminal 2 [5].

An important aspect in choosing the technology used is also the ease with which the mechanism can be manufactured, without the need for specialized training and in proximity to the field of operation (optometry). It is also important to consider the biocompatibility of the materials used, as this mechanism will be used in the immediate vicinity of patients, it is desirable that it does not affect their health in any way. One last important aspect is the possibility of recycling these devices. Choosing a metal or composite material will make it difficult to recycle the material to produce other devices [6].

Starting from the conditions listed above, several more variants of materials and manufacturing technologies have been considered. These include:

- Plastic injection—the first of the technologies considered has the disadvantage of the very high initial cost (mould cost), as well as the difficulties encountered in case of modification to the initial model [7–10]

This technological process can only be considered if it is desired to produce a very large number of components, without changing their shape [7–10].

- Selective laser sintering—this technology allows rapid modification of the model used, is compatible with elastic materials, but the prohibitive costs and special conditions of use make it unsuitable for the requested model [11–14].
- Stereolithography—this technology has several advantages, such as the relatively low price of the equipment and ease of use, while disadvantages include the high cost of the polymer and the fact that it requires ventilation installation [15–18].
- Thermoplastic extrusion—FDM technology allows the realization of prototypes in a very short time, from a very wide range of materials that have a low price and are affordable [19–22].

The wide spread of this technology has allowed for the very rapid development of both commercial solutions for depositing plastic in layers and materials. FDM technology involves the deposition of a continuous flow of material in the form of a heated filament to obtain geometric shapes, under the control of a computer system. Deposition usually occurs on the x and y axes (plane) with the increment of the Z axis after complete deposition of the material on the current layer. The thermoplastic materials used are part of an extraordinarily wide range and include Polylactic acid PLA, Acrylonitrile Butadiene Styrene ABS, Thermoplastic Polyurethane TPU, Nylon, Polyethylene terephthalate glycol PETG, and other variations of them or composite materials.

Among the presented solutions, the FDM technology corresponds in terms of cost and quality for the execution of the compliant mechanism [23].

The materials used to make the mechanism were chosen based on the mechanical characteristics, availability, and cost price: PLA, ABS and TPU. The shape of the mechanism was determined after multiple experiments over several iterations and using the pros and cons of current marked solutions. Regarding the size and stroke of the mechanism, they were determined by measuring the lowest and highest frame sizes usually encountered in the industry. Furthermore, a key determining factor of the size was the industry standards in terms of lens size before it is cut to fit the frames (between 60–70 mm). Along with this, the shape allows for easy dimensioning up or down, with regards to using FDM technology.

The shape and usability cases for the device were based on tens of years of experience in the field of optometry. For the shape and requirements for the system, feedback received from users who have employed similar systems for a number of years was considered. Since the device will come into contact directly with both the optometrist and the patients, it was very important that their feedback be the starting point for the design, and also, that ease of use was a significant factor in determining the final shape of the frame. There are no similar devices on the market in terms of the shape of the device, method of use, or technologies used to produce it. Table 1 presents several constructive solutions proposed by the authors with the characteristics described.

Table 1. Several proposed designed shapes for the compliant mechanism.

Model	Explanation
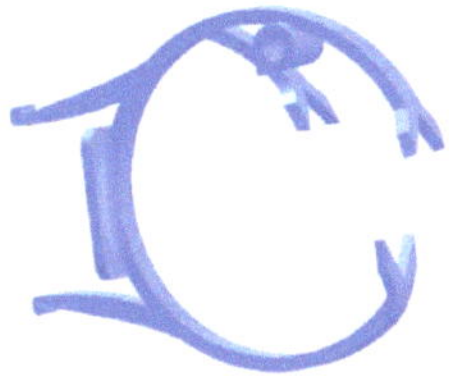	Version 1—Loosely based on a half open contour of glasses frames, the two-sided handles allow force to be applied, and thus obtain an almost vertical movement of the three prongs in the right of the picture. These three points will allow for secure fastening to the frames. The model was found lacking for multiple reasons, especially due to the fact that applying the necessary force was difficult.
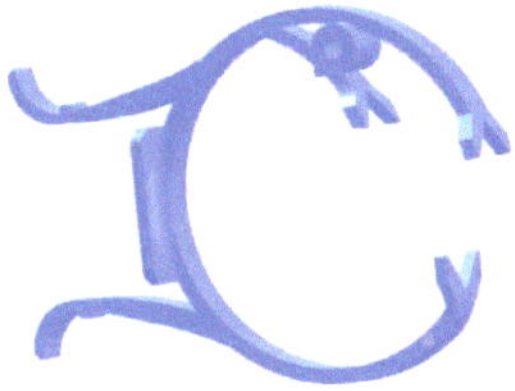	Version 2—The improved design of the handles allows force to be applied much more easily, and thus obtain a better overall behaviour. However, in this version, it was first noticed that the new support interfered with the patient, since the actual body of the marker support system pushed against the patient's face.
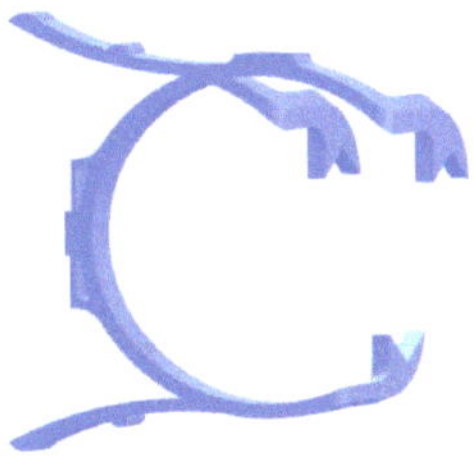	Version 3—Prongs were extended laterally to move the entire support in a plane parallel to the user's glasses, and as such, no longer pushed against the patient's face. Modifications were also made to the handles with minor improvements to the overall usability of the system.
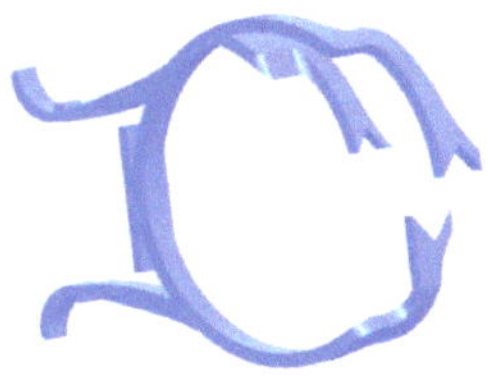	Version 4—Further improvements were made to the design, and handles were reverted to the initial profile, as the previous one was proven to fail under repeated stress in terms of both simulations and practical use.
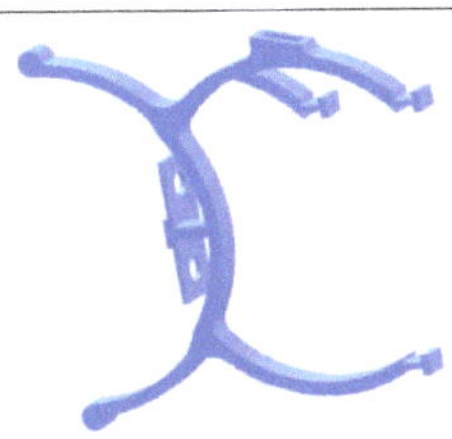	Version 5—To allow for a larger opening of the device, the orientation of the handles was changed. Furthermore, the prongs were made detachable—this is due to the technological aspects of FDM, as it allows for much better control of the settings used for each part of the frame. Furthermore, since the prongs are in direct contact with the frames, they must be coated to ensure that they do not scratch the surface.
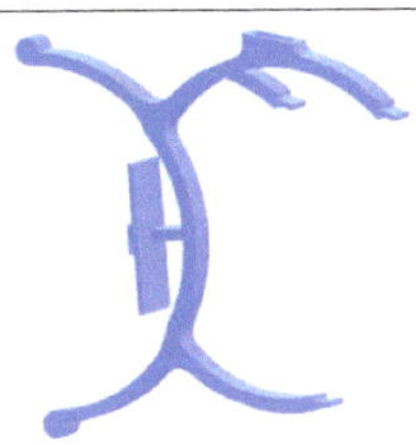	Version 6—Final version of the design, with minor modifications in terms of the retention system for prongs, infill, as well as very small dimensional changes. This is the version that has been used in the paper.

2. Finite Element Analysis of Proposed Shape

In order to predict the displacement of the proposed system and, in this sense, to choose the optimal material to realize the physical model for the given application, the designed structures were simulated using the finite element method, starting with three materials frequently used in FDM technology.

With the help of finite element method analysis, the 3D model was simulated assuming that it was divided into several smaller elements, with their size and number depending on the fineness of the meshing.

Exact numerical models should predict the mechanical behaviour of an investigated structure, but in most cases these models must be validated. To be confirmed first, the correct geometry and the corresponding characteristics of the materials used are required. Furthermore, the exactness of the values obtained by the finite element method analysis depends to a large extent on the fineness of the measurement and discretization parameters, but, at the same time, it also depends on the correct application of mechanical loads. The combination of Finite Element Analysis FEA with experimental validation of the mechanical behaviour of the compliant mechanisms investigated can be considered the most appropriate way to study, compare, and choose the optimal materials and/or manufacturing technologies for this application, and when the results of numerical and experimental methods are close, the developed structure can be validated.

In this FEM study, three thermoplastic materials were used that could be possible candidates for the marker clamp systems used in the optometric field—acrylonitrile butadiene styrene (ABS) [24–27], polylactic acid (PLA) [28–31], and thermoplastic polyurethane (TPU) [32–35], and as a medium, SolidWorks was used for the simulation. The main mechanical properties for the materials used in the study are represented in Table 2 [36–38], which are essential elements for the correctness of the results obtained by Finite Element Method FEM analysis. The main steps for performing the numerical simulation can be highlighted are the application of the material, the definition of the fixed geometries, the application of the loads, and their division into finite elements—the meshing. The following measurement parameters were used in this study:

- Mesh type: Solid Mesh
- Element Size: 1.43838 mm
- Tolerance: 0.0719189 mm
- Mesh Quality: High
- Total Nodes: 15,490
- Total Elements: 8368
- Maximum Aspect Ratio: 13,989
- % of elements with Aspect Ratio < 3: 96.5
- % of elements with Aspect Ratio > 10: 0.0956
- % of distorted elements (Jacobian): 0

Table 2. Properties of materials used in the study.

Property	ABS	PLA	TPU
Density	1.02 g/cm^3	1.252 g/cm^3	1.18 g/cm^3
Young Modulus	1.18 GPa	1.59 GPa	0.396 GPa
Poisson ratio	0.35	0.36	0.3897
Yield strength	45 MPa	70 MPa	65.85 MPa

Figure 2 shows some simulation steps and the results obtained for TPU when applying a force of 35 N, also observing the way in which the structure is deformed.

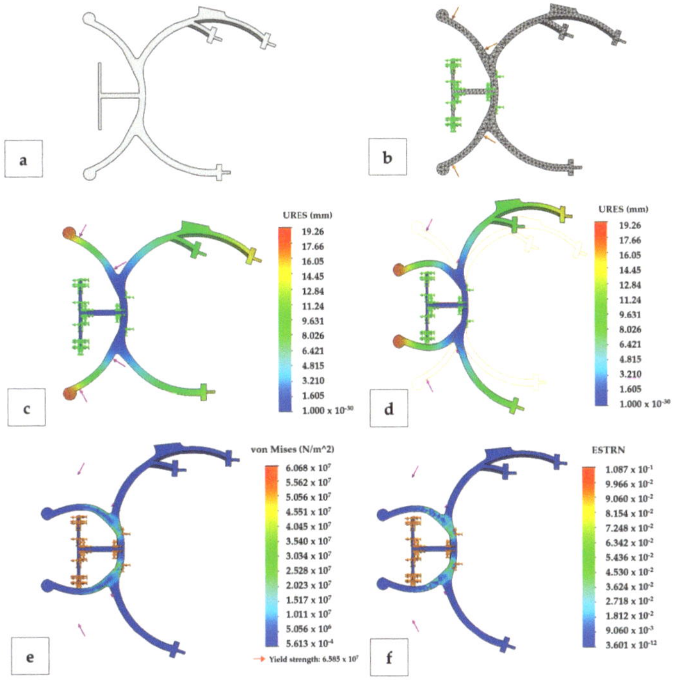

Figure 2. Some steps of FEM simulation of the TPU compliant mechanism at 35 N applied force: (**a**)-geometry model designing; (**b**)-fixing geometry, applying force and meshing; (**c**)-displacement results (undeformed model); (**d**)-displacement results (deformed model); (**e**)-Von Mises stress results; (**f**)-strain results (the arrows represent the mode of action of the force).

Figure 3 shows the results obtained for the mechanical characteristics of interest: the equivalent Von Mises stresses and the maximum opening or distance/displacement obtained between the two fastening elements. The Von Mises stresses obtained for all three investigated materials are presented in Figure 3a,c,e, and it can be observed that for the ABS material the value of Von Mises stress at 35 N exceeds the yield strength of the material. To obtain the results of the maximum opening of the compliant mechanism as a result of applying the request, it was set from SW to only display the results of the entities of interest, as shown in Figure 3b,d,f, the total distance obtained by summing the resulting displacements of the two clamping elements.

Figure 4 shows the comparative results of the displacements at the same applied force (35 N) for the three materials used in the study, clearly observing the much higher degree of deformation of the compliant mechanism of TPU, especially due to its mechanical properties being much more suitable for this application. Therefore, for the same applied force of 35 N, a maximum aperture of 27.86 mm is obtained for TPU (which corresponds to the real displacement range for the application of the compliant mechanism), a much higher value compared to those obtained for ABS and PLA—9.74 mm and 7.17 mm, respectively. Table 3 shows the simulation results obtained for the three materials studied in a certain force range (5–35 N) for the equivalent Von Mises stresses and the maximum openings of the compliant mechanism. It can be seen from the table, that at applied forces greater than 25 N, for ABS, the Von Mises stresses exceed the material yield limit, which indicates possible plastic deformation in some areas where this value is exceeded; an undesirable aspect for the application of the compliant mechanism.

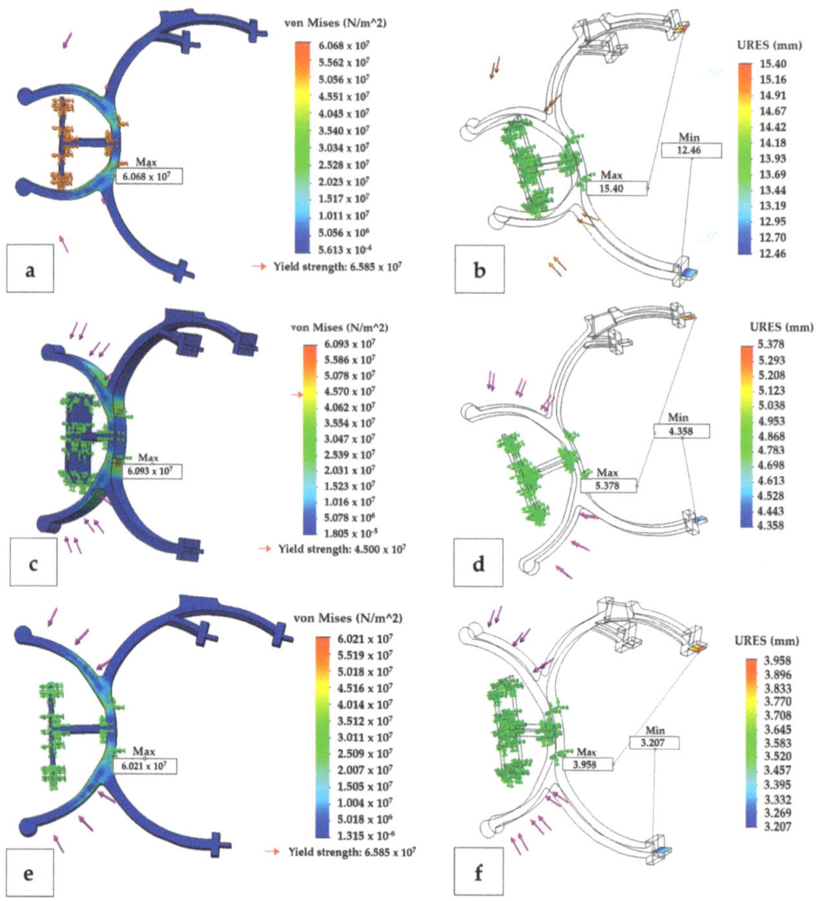

Figure 3. Comparison of obtained mechanical characteristics results for three investigated materials (35 N applied force in all cases): (**a**)-TPU mechanism Von Mises stress results; (**b**)-TPU mechanism displacement results between gripping elements; (**c**)-ABS mechanism Von Mises stress results; (**d**)-ABS mechanism displacement results between gripping elements; (**e**)-PLA mechanism Von Mises stress results; (**f**)-PLA mechanism displacement results between gripping elements.

Figure 5 shows the comparative results of the displacements of the fastening elements obtained according to the force for all three studied materials, where the much higher values for TPU of the displacements at the same applied force compared to acrylonitrile butadiene styrene and polylactic acid are clearly highlighted, to conclude that this material seems to be the most suitable candidate for the realization of the fastening systems applied in the field of clinical optometry discussed in this paper. This is due to its special mechanical properties that are manifested by increased elasticity and other important properties that recommend it for this application in the field of optometry. Between PLA and ABS, the former proved to have more suitable properties after simulation tests.

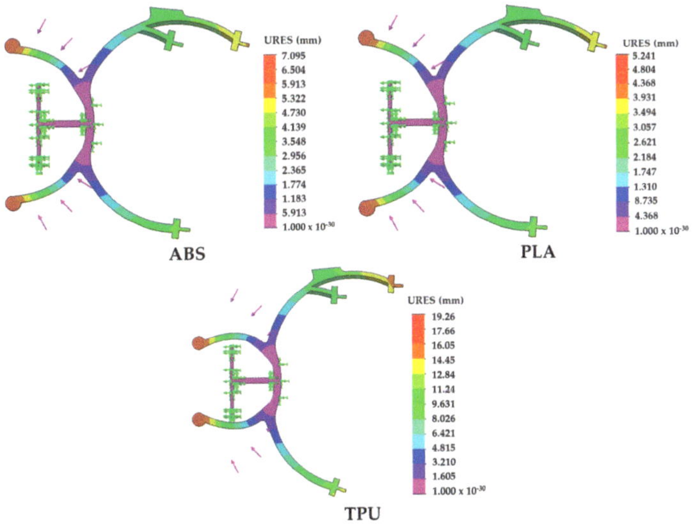

Figure 4. Comparison of resulted displacement and degree deformation at the same applied force-35 N for all investigated materials.

Table 3. Obtained results for Von Mises stress and displacement between gripping elements.

F (N)	TPU (σ_y = 65.85 MPa)		ABS (σ_y = 45 MPa)		PLA (σ_y = 70 MPa)	
	y_{max} [mm]	σ_{max} [MPa]	y_{max} [mm]	σ_{max} [MPa]	y_{max} [mm]	σ_{max} [MPa]
5	4.03	8.4	1.35	8.35	1.03	8.3
10	8.16	17.16	2.72	16.84	2.01	16.72
15	12.32	26.11	4.11	25.47	3.03	25.25
20	16.42	35.07	5.51	34.21	4.05	33.87
25	20.4	43.87	6.91	43.05	5.09	42.58
30	24.23	52.45	8.32	51.96	6.12	51.36
35	27.86	60.68	9.74	60.93	7.17	60.21

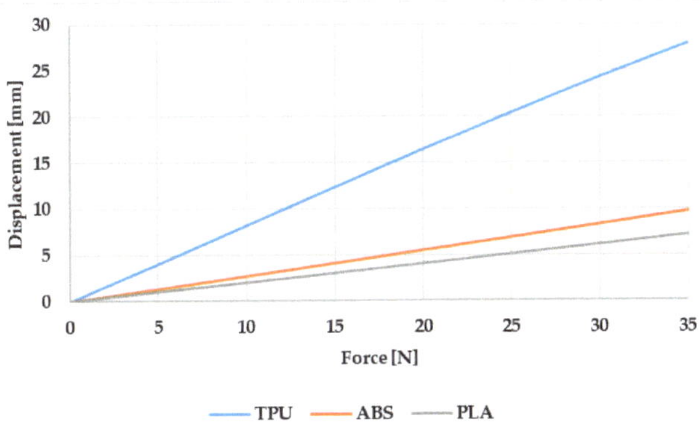

Figure 5. Comparison of force-displacement characteristics for investigated materials.

Figure 6 shows the simulation results (35 N applied force) for a constructive variant consisting of four fastening elements, which can be used to fasten circular glasses. In this case, a maximum opening between the outer fasteners of 29.16 mm is obtained at an applied force of 35 N. In both constructive cases (with three and four gripping elements), following the FEM analysis, the most suitable material for the given application is TPU, where the closest displacement compared to the desired displacement is obtained according to theoretical considerations.

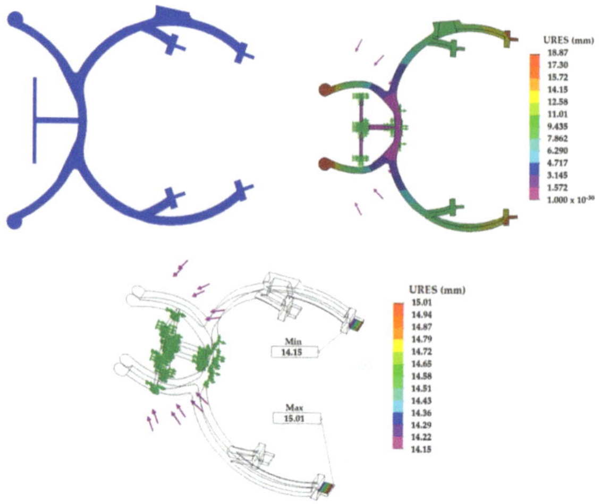

Figure 6. Obtained results for compliant mechanism with four gripping elements.

3. Physically Developed Prototype of Mechanism

The mechanism was manufactured using FDM technology from PLA, ABS, and TPU (Figure 7). When using each material, the particularities of each thermoplastic used were considered. No special problems were encountered in the realization of the three variants, but noticeable differences were observed between the times necessary to print the mechanisms. Thus, the TPU material is the most expensive in terms of time, being necessary to use it at very low speeds (10–20 mm/s-Figure 8), compared to PLA/ABS (30–35 mm/s), the results being similar in terms of aesthetics.

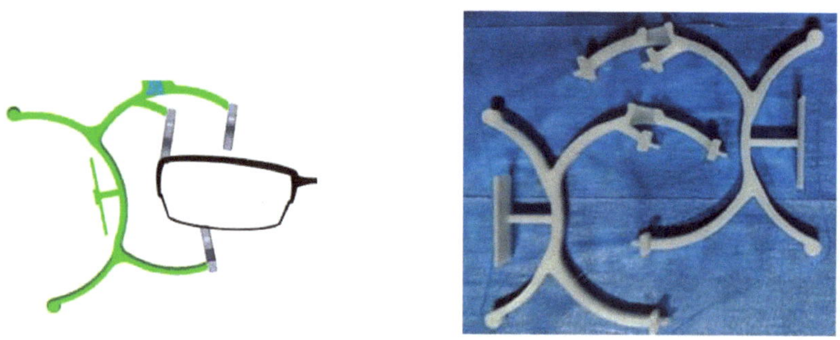

Figure 7. Principle of operation and PLA manufactured compliant mechanism.

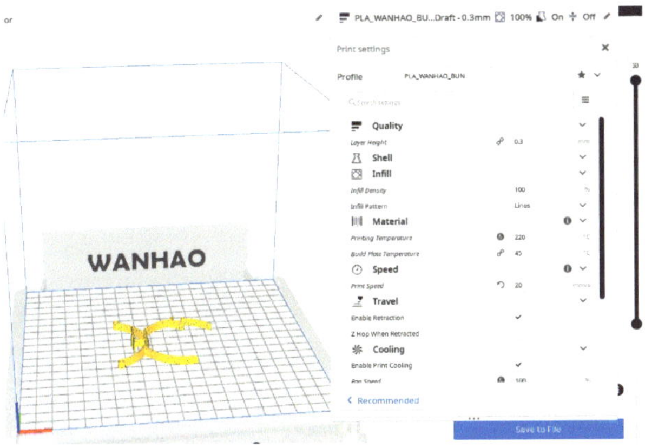

Figure 8. Working parameters used for compliant mechanism.

As expected from the point of view of the use of the materials presented, the differences between the three are obvious. For the following conclusions, a series of tests were performed with the help of human users. Their automatic testing was performed in the next part of the paper.

The PLA material variants used give way after several uses, but are the easiest to obtain and, from an aesthetic point of view, they correspond to the requirements. The approximate weight obtained is 4 g.

The ABS material presents, as expected, problems in terms of realization, it being necessary to add a layer of sacrifice. The results are similar to those obtained for PLA: although appropriate from an aesthetic point of view and with a very wide range of colours, the pieces made do not correspond, in terms of elasticity, to the requirements and give way after several uses.

Thermoplastic polyurethane (TPU)—from the variants used and commercially available, the NinjaTek Armadillo variant was chosen, which was also used for the simulations presented above [38]. Although it presents a series of challenges in terms of use in the FDM process, this material is mechanically the most suitable, obtaining the desired displacements for the forces that can be exerted during use by a human user.

Among the materials used, the best results were obtained for TPU, with the disadvantage of having less pleasant surfaces from an aesthetic point of view, and with some difficulties in printing the parts. This contradicts some of the conditions imposed at the beginning of the work—the possibility of realizing these mechanisms without a specialized training, with the help of common 3D printers. This material is also biocompatible, as stated by the manufacturer.

4. Testing of Manufactured Device

In order to test and validate the structures made by FDM technology, but also to compare the results obtained by simulation with the results of the experimental model, a physical system was developed that simulated the functioning of the proposed mechanisms for the given application. The experimental stand proposed in the paper presents the possibility of fixing the tested part in a support that allows its displacement, especially on the X axis and the rotation around the Z axis of the compliant mechanism. The testing rig was specially made for the tests and is not part of any patent or technical solution. Its purpose was to determine if the mechanism could be used for a reasonable number of times, less than a couple hundred, without it breaking or losing its mechanical characteristics, and testing was continuously performed.

However, the part was not fixed on any axis; the assembly was made with high tolerances. At each of the moving ends of the mechanism, end-of-travel sensors were mounted, as shown, for clarity, as mechanical microswitches in the diagram in Figure 9, but optical sensors in the stand were made. Actuation was conducted with the help of two linear pneumatic motors with double action (Figure 10), dimensioned so as to produce a force of, at most, 35 N at the working pressure (3 bar). The two motors were mounted in opposition on the same Y axis of the system, in the direction of the red arrows in Figure 9. The movement of the two motors simultaneously occurred, according to the proposed control algorithm.

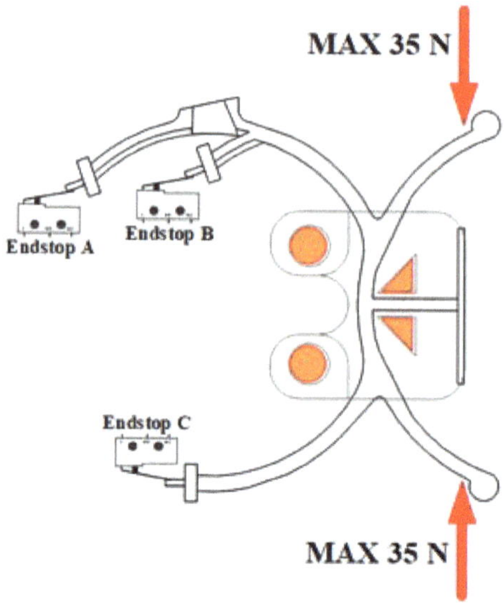

Figure 9. Principle schematics of testing.

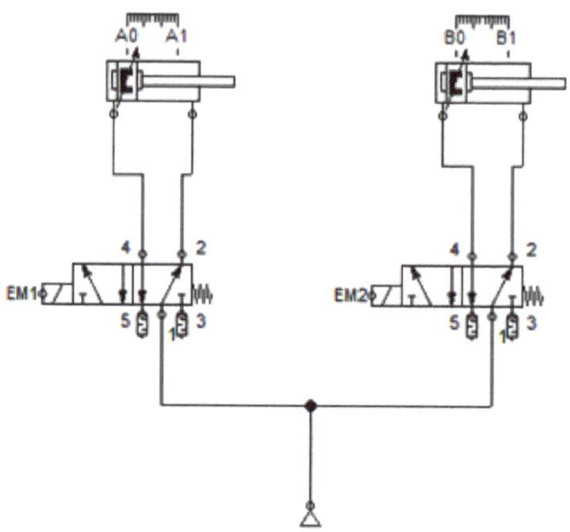

Figure 10. Pneumatic actuation schematics.

The control and monitoring of the system was conducted with the help of an electronic system based on an ESP microcontroller, together with the signal adaptation electronics necessary for the interface with the distributors and limit switches used.

Figure 11 shows a schematic diagram of the algorithm implemented for control.

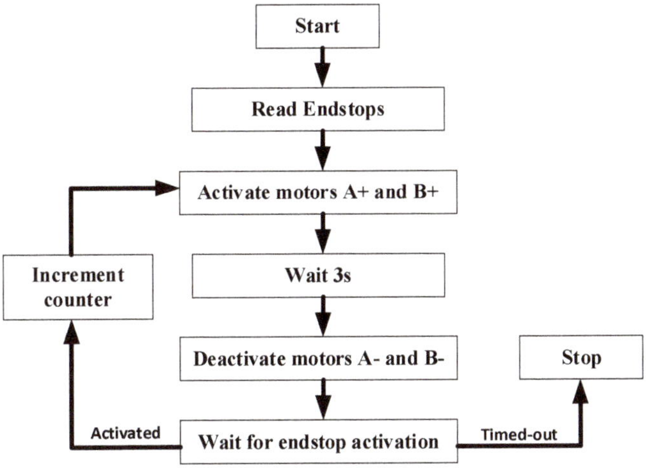

Figure 11. Control algorithm schematics.

Figure 12a shows the complete scheme of the system made for testing the parts. A simple PC-level application was developed to control the application. This opens a bidirectional TCP port and allows for the initiation of commands and the reception of data from the limit switches mounted on the construction. The advance and withdrawal strokes along with the signals from the end-of-travel sensors were counted at the controller level and transmitted to the PC.

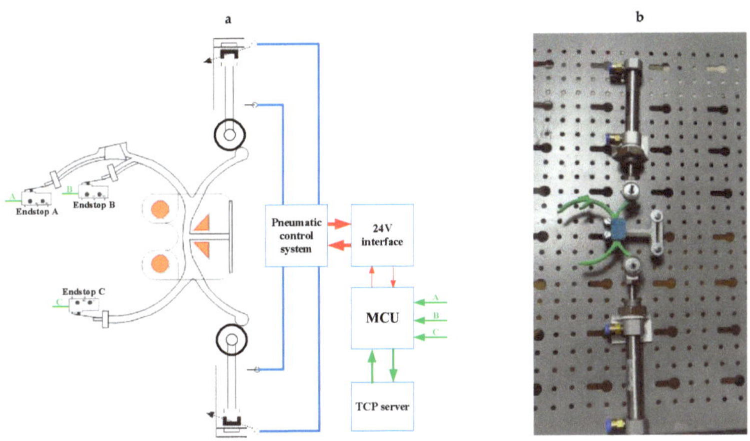

Figure 12. (**a**)—Control schematics; (**b**)—Real system.

Figure 12b shows an overview of the test stand made for testing this solution and obtained preliminary results to confirm those obtained by the simulation. It contains the elements presented above and works according to those described.

As expected, the system poorly performs for both ABS and PLA, with minimal elasticity of the parts, and they fail after only a few uses. TPU parts, however, perform generally better, as tested, with no obvious issues to the mechanism after a few tries.

5. Conclusions

This paper presents the the right choice of materials, a finite element analysis simulation, technologies, and the realization and testing of mechanisms to be used in the field of optometry. Following the research, the chosen thermoplastic polyurethane (TPU) material proved to be the most suitable, both in terms of elastic properties, biocompatibility, the possibility of recycling materials, and all criteria stated at the beginning of the paper. From a scientific standpoint, the model is set to serve as part of a low-cost, low-maintenance system with a reasonable error parameter needed for custom-built lenses for users with specific needs. This is set to lower the cost of such procedures, which is currently high, and is also expected to assist in giving better medical care to a larger array of individuals.

In the future, we want to test this mechanism in a complete set, but also perform tests with as many patients as possible, so that the possible problems related to the use and implementation of the mechanism described in this paper can be determined and solved.

Author Contributions: Conceptualization, V.C. and E.M.; methodology, V.C. and B.G.; software, V.C. and B.G.; validation, E.M. and D.B.; formal analysis, E.M. and D.B.; investigation, D.B. and V.C.; resources, B.G. and E.M.; writing—original draft preparation, V.C., E.M., D.B. and B.G.; writing—review and editing V.C., E.M., D.B. and B.G. All authors have read and agreed to the published version of the manuscript.

Funding: This research received no external funding.

Institutional Review Board Statement: Not applicable.

Informed Consent Statement: Not applicable.

Data Availability Statement: Not applicable.

Conflicts of Interest: The authors declare no conflict of interest.

References

1. Nilsen, T.; Hermann, M.; Eriksen, C.; Dagfinrud, H.; Mowinckel, P.; Kjeken, I. Grip force and pinch grip in an adult population Reference values and factors associated with grip force. *Scand. J. Occup. Ther.* **2011**, *19*, 288–296. [CrossRef]
2. VisionFit Dispensing System™ (VFDS). Available online: https://www.luzerneoptical.com/vfds-visionfit-dispensing-system html (accessed on 6 January 2023).
3. What Is OptikamPad? Available online: https://www.optikam.com/ (accessed on 6 January 2023).
4. EssilorPRO. Available online: https://www.essilorpro.com/ (accessed on 6 January 2023).
5. ZEISS i.Terminal 2. Available online: https://www.zeiss.com/vision-care/int/ecp/products/instruments-technology/zeiss-i terminal-2.html (accessed on 6 January 2023).
6. Thompson, M.; Moroni, G.; Vaneker, T.; Fadel, G.; Campbell, R.; Gibson, I.; Bernard, A.; Schulz, J.; Graf, P.; Ahuja, B.; et al. Design for Additive Manufacturing: Trends, opportunities, considerations, and constraints. *CIRP Ann.* **2016**, *65*, 737–760. [CrossRef]
7. Farooque, R.; Asjad, M.; Rizvi, S. A current state of art applied to injection moulding manufacturing process—A review. *Mater Today Proc.* **2021**, *43*, 441–446. [CrossRef]
8. Singh, G.; Verma, A. A Brief Review on injection moulding manufacturing process. *Mater. Today Proc.* **2017**, *4*, 1423–1433 [CrossRef]
9. Hamidi, M.F.F.A.; Harun, W.S.W.; Samykano, M.; Ghani, S.A.C.; Ghazalli, Z.; Ahmad, F.; Sulon, A.B. A review of biocompatible metal injection moulding process parameters for biomedical applications. *Mater. Sci. Eng. C* **2017**, *78*, 1263–1276. [CrossRef]
10. Dehghan-Manshadi, A.; Yu, P.; Dargush, M.; Stjohn, D.; Qian, M. Metal injection moulding of surgical tools, biomaterials and medical devices: A review. *Powder Technol.* **2020**, *364*, 189–204. [CrossRef]
11. Mazzoli, A. Selective laser sintering in biomedical engineering. *Med. Biol. Eng. Comput.* **2013**, *51*, 245–256. [CrossRef]
12. Kumar, S. Selective laser sintering: A qualitative and objective approach. *JOM* **2003**, *55*, 43–47. [CrossRef]
13. Schmidt, M.; Pohle, D.; Rechtenwald, T. Selective Laser Sintering of PEEK. *CIRP Ann.* **2007**, *56*, 205–208. [CrossRef]
14. Olakanmi, E.; Cochrane, R.; Dalgarno, K. A review on selective laser sintering/melting (SLS/SLM) of aluminium alloy powders Processing, microstructure, and properties. *Prog. Mater. Sci.* **2015**, *74*, 401–477. [CrossRef]
15. León-Cabezas, M.; Martínez-García, A.; Varela-Gandía, F. Innovative advances in additive manufactured moulds for short plastic injection series. *Procedia Manuf.* **2017**, *13*, 732–737. [CrossRef]
16. Medellin, A.; Du, W.; Miao, G.; Zou, J.; Pei, Z.; Ma, C. Vat Photopolymerization 3D Printing of Nanocomposites: A Literature Review. *J. Micro Nano-Manuf.* **2019**, *7*, 031006. [CrossRef]
17. Aduba, D.C., Jr.; Margaretta, E.D.; Marnot, A.E.; Heifferon, K.V.; Surbey, W.R.; Chartrain, N.A.; Whittington, A.R.; Long, T.E. Williams, C.B. Vat photopolymerization 3D printing of acid-cleavable PEG-methacrylate networks for biomaterial applications *Mater. Today Commun.* **2019**, *19*, 204–211. [CrossRef]
18. Chartrain, N.A.; Williams, C.B.; Whittington, A.R. A review on fabricating tissue scaffolds using vat photopolymerization. *Acta Biomater.* **2018**, *74*, 90–111. [CrossRef]

19. Dhinakaran, V.; Manoj Kumar, K.; Bupathi Ram, P.; Ravichandran, M.; Vinayagamoorthy, M. A review on recent advancements in fused deposition modelling. *Mater. Today Proc.* **2020**, *27*, 752–756. [CrossRef]
20. Parulski, C.; Jennotte, O.; Lechanteur, A.; Evrard, B. Challenges of fused deposition modeling 3D printing in pharmaceutical applications: Where are we now? *Adv. Drug Deliv. Rev.* **2021**, *175*, 113810. [CrossRef]
21. Cailleaux, S.; Sanchez-Ballester, N.M.; Gueche, Y.A.; Bataille, B.; Soulairol, I. Fused Deposition Modeling (FDM), the new asset for the production of tailored medicines. *J. Control. Release* **2021**, *330*, 821–841. [CrossRef]
22. Bakır, A.A.; Atik, R.; Özerinç, S. Mechanical properties of thermoplastic parts produced by fused deposition modeling: A review. *Rapid Prototyp. J.* **2021**, *27*, 537–561. [CrossRef]
23. Doshi, M.; Mahale, A.; Kumar Singh, S.; Deshmukh, S. Printing parameters and materials affecting mechanical properties of FDM-3D printed Parts: Perspective and prospects. *Mater. Today Proc.* **2022**, *50*, 2269–2275. [CrossRef]
24. Rezaeian, P.; Ayatollahi, M.R.; Nabavi-Kivi, A.; Razavi SM, J. Effect of printing speed on tensile and fracture behavior of ABS specimens produced by fused deposition modelling. *Eng. Fract. Mech.* **2022**, *266*, 108393. [CrossRef]
25. Azadi, M.; Dadashi, A.; Dezianian, S.; Kianifar, M.; Torkaman, S.; Chiyani, M. High-cycle bending fatigue properties of additive-manufactured ABS and PLA polymers fabricated by fused deposition modeling 3D-printing. *Forces Mech.* **2021**, *3*, 100016. [CrossRef]
26. Peterson, A.M. Review of acrylonitrile butadiene styrene in fused filament fabrication: A plastics engineering-focused perspective. *Addit. Manuf.* **2019**, *27*, 363–371. [CrossRef]
27. Vidakis, N. Sustainable additive manufacturing: Mechanical response of acrylonitrile-butadiene-styrene over multiple recycling processes. *Sustainability* **2020**, *12*, 3568. [CrossRef]
28. Singhvi, M.S.; Zinjarde, S.S.; Gokhale, D.V. Polylactic acid: Synthesis and biomedical applications. *J. Appl. Microbiol.* **2019**, *127*, 1612–1626. [CrossRef]
29. Li, G.; Zhao, M.; Xu, F.; Yang, B.; Li, X.; Meng, X.; Teng, L.; Sun, F.; Li, Y. Synthesis and biological application of polylactic acid. *Molecules* **2020**, *25*, 5023. [CrossRef]
30. Casalini, T.; Rossi, F.; Castrovinci, A.; Perale, G. A Perspective on Polylactic Acid-Based Polymers Use for Nanoparticles Synthesis and Applications. *Front. Bioeng. Biotechnol.* **2019**, *7*, 259. [CrossRef]
31. Hamad, K.; Kaseem, M.; Ayyoob, M.; Joo, J.; Deri, F. Polylactic acid blends: The future of green, light and tough. *Prog. Polym. Sci.* **2018**, *85*, 83–127. [CrossRef]
32. Xiao, J.; Gao, Y. The manufacture of 3D printing of medical grade TPU. *Prog. Addit. Manuf.* **2017**, *2*, 117–123. [CrossRef]
33. Verstraete, G.; Samaro, A.; Grymonpré, W.; Vanhoorne, V.; Van Snick, B.; Boone, M.N.; Hellemans, T.; Van Hoorebeke, L.; Remon, J.P.; Vervaet, C. 3D printing of high drug loaded dosage forms using thermoplastic polyurethanes. *Int. J. Pharm.* **2018**, *536*, 318–325. [CrossRef]
34. Harris, C.G.; Jursik, N.J.; Rochefort, W.E.; Walker, T.W. Additive Manufacturing with Soft TPU—Adhesion Strength in Multimaterial Flexible Joints. *Front. Mech. Eng.* **2019**, *5*, 37. [CrossRef]
35. De la Rosa, S.; Mayuet, P.F.; Méndez Salgueiro, J.R.; Rodríguez-Parada, L. Design of Customized TPU Lattice Structures for Additive Manufacturing: Influence on the Functional Properties in Elastic Products. *Polymers* **2021**, *13*, 4341. [CrossRef]
36. Moraru, E. Research on the Realization of Dental Prostheses by Selective Laser Deposition and Other Additive Technologies. Ph.D. Thesis, Politehnica University of Bucharest, Bucharest, Romania, 2021. (In Romanian).
37. Besnea, D.; Rizescu, C.I.; Rizescu, D.; Comeaga, D.; Ciobanu, R.; Moraru, E. Study of deflection behaviour of 3D printed leaf springs. In Proceedings of the 8th International Conference on Advanced Concepts in Mechanical Engineering, Iasi, Romania, 7–8 June 2018; Volume 444, p. 042008.
38. Armadillo Technical Data Sheet. Available online: https://ninjatek.com/shop/armadillo/ (accessed on 6 January 2023).

applied sciences

MDPI

Article

Examining Gait Characteristics in People with Osteoporosis Utilizing a Non-Wheeled Smart Walker through Spatiotemporal Analysis

Nazia Ejaz [1,2], Saad Jawaid Khan [3,*], Fahad Azim [1], Mehwish Faiz [3], Emil Teuțan [4], Alin Pleșa [4], Alexandru Ianosi-Andreeva-Dimitrova [4] and Sergiu-Dan Stan [4,*]

1 Department of Electrical Engineering, Ziauddin University, Karachi 74600, Pakistan; nazia_ejaz94@yahoo.com (N.E.); fahad.azim@zu.edu.pk (F.A.)
2 Department of Biomedical Engineering, Balochistan University of Engineering & Technology, Khuzdar 89100, Pakistan
3 Department of Biomedical Engineering, Ziauddin University, Karachi 74600, Pakistan; mehwish.faiz@zu.edu.pk
4 Department of Mechatronics and Machine Dynamics, Technical University of Cluj-Napoca, 400114 Cluj-Napoca, Romania; emil.teutan@mdm.utcluj.ro (E.T.); alin.plesa@mdm.utcluj.ro (A.P.); alexandru.ianosi@mdm.utcluj.ro (A.I.-A.-D.)
* Correspondence: sj.khan@zu.edu.pk (S.J.K.); sergiu.stan@mdm.utcluj.ro (S.-D.S.)

Abstract: Fragility fractures, caused by low-energy trauma, are a significant global health concern, with 158 million people aged 50 and over at risk. Hip fractures, a common issue in elderly patients, are often linked to underlying conditions such as osteoporosis. This study proposed a cost-effective solution using a non-wheeled smart walker with load sensors to measure gait parameters, addressing the high cost of traditional gait analysis equipment, the prototype used PASCO load cells PS2200 for force measurement, eliminating the need for Arduino UNO or microcontroller-based hardware. A lightweight amplifier PS2198 amplified the signal, which was transmitted via USB to a personal computer. PASCO capstone software was used for data recording and visualization. The smart walker was tested on forty volunteers divided into two equal groups: those with osteoporosis and those without, by performing a 10 m walk test three times. ANOVA comparing spatiotemporal parameters (TSPs) of the two participant groups ($\alpha = 0.05$) showed that significant differences lay in terms of time taken to complete the walk test ($p < 0.01$), left step length ($p = 0.03$), walking speed ($p = 0.02$), and stride length ($p < 0.02$). The results indicate that this smart walker is a reliable tool for assessing gait patterns in individuals with osteoporosis. The proposed system can be an alternative for time consuming and costly methods such as motion capture, and for socially stigmatizing devices such as exoskeletons. It can also be used further to identify risk factors of osteoporosis.

Keywords: fracture prevention; bone health; mobility aid geriatric care; spatiotemporal analysis; osteoporotic fractures; hip fracture; elderly healthcare; biomechanical assessment; fall prevention; osteoporosis management; physical therapy; musculoskeletal disorders; aging population; medical technology; clinical research; bone density; patient rehabilitation; functional mobility; osteoporosis diagnosis

1. Introduction

Osteoporosis is a medical condition distinguished by a reduction in bone mineral density. It can be coupled with a decline in muscle mass and an increase in the deposition of adipose tissue. These physiological alterations can influence an individual's gait and equilibrium, increasing their vulnerability to falls and fractures [1]. The decrease in bone density in osteoporosis causes injury to the hip joint by exposing it to heightened stress levels. This phenomenon is notably prevalent in postmenopausal females. The increased stress makes seemingly healthy hip joints susceptible to osteoarthritis through perturbations to the typical patterns of gait and balance [2].

While conventional methods for assessing gait disturbances and fear of falling in persons with bone diseases exist, they often necessitate manual patient evaluations, which can be cumbersome for both the patient and the clinician. For instance, the dual cognitive task test can gauge gait abnormalities in individuals afflicted with osteoporosis and a fear of falling [3], while the ten-meter test assesses the impact of training programs on balance, gait velocity, and muscle strength in people with osteoporosis [4]. However, these manual assessments mandate specialized testing facilities and trained therapists to administer them, rendering them impractical in various settings.

To address these challenges, alternative automated systems have emerged to conduct gait analysis and assessments [5]. These systems encompass a wide array of technologies, including motion capture systems [6,7], and video cameras [8]. While undeniably effective in suitable contexts with the requisite infrastructure and trained personnel, these methods are not universally accessible or convenient.

Another avenue involves the utilization of sensors, such as inertial measurement units (IMUs) [9], wearable sensors [10], or insole foot pressure sensors and accelerometers [11,12]. These sensors offer the advantage of portability and can be employed in diverse environments. However, they necessitate attachment to specific body locations, which may not always be convenient or comfortable for the user.

A promising solution to these challenges lies in the integration of gait-monitoring sensors into mobility aids commonly used by individuals, such as rollators [13–15], and canes [16,17]. This innovative approach ensures that gait analysis is accessible irrespective of location or time, without requiring specific body attachments. Nonetheless, it is essential to note that this method may yield approximated gait information and, consequently, is susceptible to a margin of error compared to more intricate systems [18].

Moreover, the current focus primarily gravitates towards rollators, often equipped with wheel encoders to estimate the distance covered. However, an often-overlooked segment of the population consists of users with pronounced instability, rendering rollators impractical and even hazardous during routine activities or gait monitoring. Consequently, non-wheeled walkers emerge as a pertinent alternative in facilitating gait analysis for individuals grappling with high instability and an aversion to the risks associated with traditional rollators.

Numerous studies have been conducted to analyze gait through different techniques. The four common techniques including the use of a cane, robotic walker, pick up standard walker, and smart walker/rollator are presented in Table 1.

Table 1. Related work based on robotic walkers, canes, wheeled walkers, and standard walkers.

Robotic Walkers					
Reference	**Technology**	**Methods**	**Results**	**Limitation**	**Year**
[19]	Mobility Assistance Robotic rollator	Data was collected by using a Laser range finder	Detected gait phases	Users needed to wear fitted clothes	2014
[20]	Assistive Robot	A proximity Sensor was used by a robotic walker to measure the distance between the user's leg and the robot.	Controlled forward walking speed of the robot according to distance between the user and robot.	Only distance and walking speed were detected.	2018
[21]	Robotic Walker; Walk-IT	Multi-camera and multimodal dataset was used for biomechanical analysis.	Biomechanical analysis of posture and gait, pose estimation, and human gait detection and tracking algorithm.	Need to wear full body motion tracking system.	2022

Table 1. *Cont.*

Canes					
Reference	**Technology**	**Methods**	**Results**	**Limitation**	**Year**
[16]	Cane	A Force sensor was attached to measure the load on the cane.	Continuously measurement using weight bearing during walking	No temporal-spatial gait parameters were estimated in this study.	2019
[22]	Cane Robot	Laser range finders were used to detect the user's leg motion.	Spatiotemporal gait parameters were measured	Users needed to wear tight pants or short skirts during monitoring.	2022
Wheeled Walkers					
Reference	**Technology**	**Method**	**Results**	**Limitation**	**Year**
[14]	i-Walker Platform	Force sensors were embedded on handlebars of the walker.	Extracted spatiotemporal gait parameters.	The user needed to put a mass of at least 3 kg on the walker handlebars for use	2015
[23]	Smart Walker	Gait monitoring by using feet position and orientation by using ISIR's smart walker prototype with Active depth sensor.	Spatial patterns are reported in this study by using a camera depth sensor without markers.	Spatiotemporal parameters were not reported in this study.	2015
[24]	Wheeled Walker	Microwave Doppler radars are embedded in the four wheels of the walker.	Gait velocity estimation for normal and abnormal gait.	Important gait parameters for diagnosis of the user's condition are not the scope of this study for instance cadence, step length, etc.	2015
[18]	i-Walker Platform	Embedded force sensors in handlebars of the walker.	Estimated force difference of handlebar sensors during walking	This system was interfaced with the optotrack system and a treadmill, so it needed a confined environment for operation.	2016
[25]	Smart Rollator, i-Walker	Data of volunteers using a smart rollator based on a force sensor, an accelerometer, and a gyroscope was classified using machine learning.	Found distinct walking-age groups according to walking speed, the forces exerted by the individual on the i-Walker.	For assessment only two parameters were known i.e., walking speed and force.	2018
[26]	Smart Walker	Smart Walker based on functionalities sit-stand assistance, navigation system, and obstacle detection with gait monitoring.	The gait parameters determined by smart walker and GaitRite were concurrently validated.	This walker only determined temporal gait parameters and extraction of spatial gait parameters are not in the scope of this system.	2019
[27]	Smart Rollator Walk-IT	Open-source modular-based rollator for gait monitoring and support. It included force sensors, encoders in the wheel, and light detection and ranging sensors.	Assessment of spatiotemporal gait parameters by leg speed information and weight bearing of users.	The main draw of this device was that it needed users' leg visibility during rollator use due to a laser-based gait analysis system. Walk-IT also encountered visibility issues when it came to tracking steps, a crucial element for gait assessment.	2022

Table 1. *Cont.*

Standard Walker					
Reference	**Technology**	**Method**	**Results**	**Limitation**	**Year**
[28]	Pick up standard walker	In this study force sensors, light detection and ranging sensors were embedded in the walker's legs.	Force unbalance on the walker's leg and motor incoordination was estimated.	Spatiotemporal gait parameters were not in the scope of this study.	2018

While assessing rehabilitative devices and identifying functional limits resulting from pathologies, three-dimensional instrumented gait analysis is a useful technique. Typical components of gait analysis include analysis of spatiotemporal parameters, joint kinetics (moments and power), kinematics (joint angles and ranges of motion), and ground reaction force analysis [29]. Research in gait analysis has been limited by focusing on specific parameters such as walking speed, and spatiotemporal parameters [23,25,26]. These parameters provide valuable insights into individual gait pattern s [30] but only represent a portion of the multifaceted domain. Walkers have been used to measure temporal, and spatial parameters [26], but often interconnected with other systems like GaitRite or treadmills, limiting their applicability to controlled environments. Alternative solutions such as the cane robot [22], Robotic walker Walk-IT [21], and smart rollator walker [19] have been employed to assess gait parameters, but they impose certain prerequisites on participants, such as wearing tight-fitting clothing or short skirts for enhanced leg movement visibility. Other devices such as the JARoW [31], i-Walker [32], and FriWalk robotic walker [33] have also been proposed and offer a good range of sensory and motor applications [34]. However, these devices are either too expensive for a developing country end-user or are too complicated to be operated by the user without the help of a specialist.

In response to these limitations, the present study endeavors to fill the gap by introducing a smart walker specifically designed to facilitate a detailed gait analysis. The smart walker allows for analysis of spatiotemporal gait parameters and offers users valuable support while minimizing the risk of fall-related injuries, a concern often associated with traditional wheeled walkers. The design of the walker places minimal weight-bearing demands on the user, making it suitable for individuals with walking disabilities undergoing rehabilitation treatment using standard walkers.

To assess the device's effectiveness, we conducted a pilot study involving 40 participants in an urban setting. The study included a detailed gait analysis of differences between individuals with and without osteoporosis to validate the proposed smart walkers' utility in people with osteoporosis. Our findings show that the benefits of the smart walker extend beyond its functional capabilities. The lack of specific attire during gait monitoring promotes greater convenience and ease of use. Specific infrastructure, such as treadmills or video cameras, is not required for its operation. This makes it suitable for a wide range of clinical and healthcare settings, including rehabilitation centers, homes, and outdoor environments.

Notably, the versatility of this developed smart walker extends beyond its functional capabilities; it does not depend on any specific infrastructure, such as treadmills or video cameras, for its operation. This feature significantly enhances its suitability for a wide range of clinical and healthcare settings, including rehabilitation centers, homes, and outdoor environments, effectively eliminating the need for participants to wear specific attire during gait monitoring, thereby promoting greater convenience and ease of use.

2. Materials and Methods

A smart walker prototype was designed to facilitate the monitoring of gait patterns in people with osteoporosis during the rehabilitation process. The prototype featured onboard force sensors integrated into the walking aid. These sensors enabled the acquisition of spatiotemporal gait parameters, including walking speed, cadence, step length, step time, stride time, and stride length. The prototype's design aimed to obviate the need for participants to wear external sensors or rely on specialized equipment such as treadmills, electronic walkways, or post-processing-dependent video cameras.

The prototype was tested on 40 volunteers, comprising 20 healthy elderly individuals and 20 older individuals diagnosed with osteoporosis. The study design was quasi-experimental, where a physiotherapist administered a standardized 10 m walk test, systematically. Spatiotemporal parameters were acquired through the smart walker including the time of walk, walking speed, cadence, step length, step time, stride time, and stride length.

Figure 1 shows Smart Walker prototype equipped with PS2200 Force Sensors. In total, four force sensors were attached on walkers legs including Force sensor on rear right side (**Fs***RRs*),Force Sensor on rear left side (**Fs***RLs*), Force Sensor on front left side (**Fs***FLs*), and Force Sensor on front right side (**Fs***FRs*).The developed prototype smart walker with the positions of sensors and electronic components labelled, walker with on board sensors, providing a visual representation of the device that was used to collect data in this study. A walker made up of aluminum body and soft rubber pads on the handlebars was utilized to assist people with osteoporosis in maintaining gait balance, stability and support during their rehabilitation process. We equipped this commercially available walker with four sensors, which were placed at the front and rear legs of the walker to measure the upper limb forces during walking. The sensors were embedded at a distance of 0.7112 m (28 inches) away from the handgrips to avoid damage from overloading. PASCO load cells PS2200 were used as a sensor in this prototype, which measured forces in all directions, eliminating the need for Arduino UNO or microcontroller-based hardware for data transmission. A lightweight load cell amplifier PS2198 was used to amplify the sensor signal, which was then transmitted to a personal computer via USB interface. The sensor signal amplifier PS2198 and USB interface PS2100 are light weight and easily travel with handheld data loggers. For data recording and visualization, PASCO capstone software v 2.0 (free trial) was used, displaying a graph of forces of right and left hands on the handlebars of walkers versus time of the walk. The system is wired but this cannot affect the measurements due to the Well-fitted sockets (six-pin mini-DIN jacks) of amplifier and USB interface which connects walker sensors to personal computer for data recording. Due to wired connections, the current design allowed users to walk up to 15 m. To record gait daily or weekly the user at home needs to setup the hardware and software as follows:

Hardware setup:

i. Connect four separate load cells to the input ports of the amplifier.
ii. Connect the cable of the load cell amplifier to a PASPORT interface.
iii. Connect the PASPORT interface to Personal Computer USB port.

Software setup (Data studio):

i. Once you connect the load cell amplifier to the computer via a PASPORT interface, the PASPortal window will open automatically as shown in Figure 2.
ii. Select launch Data Studio in PASPortal window.
iii. Click 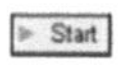

to begin data collection.

Users can save recorded data and can share it with therapist electronically for gait assessment. After recording data, the user can disconnect the amplifier and USB interface from sensor to use walker for gait support and rehabilitation every time and everywhere.

The software setup image shown in Figure 2 is taken from https://www.conatex.be/media/manuals/BAEN/BLEN_1091161.pdf source (accessed on 1 October 2023).

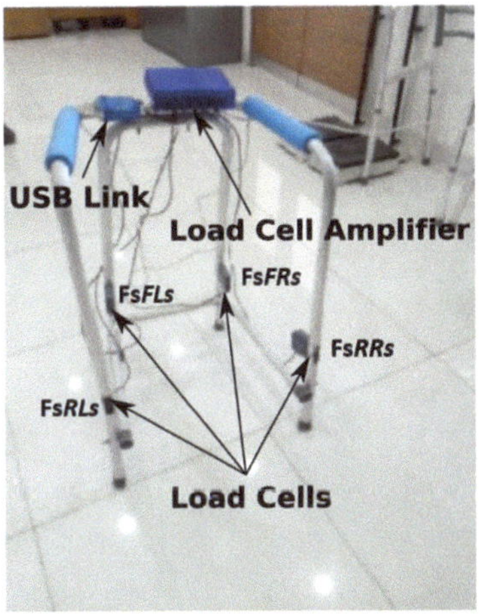

Figure 1. Smart Walker with on board sensors.

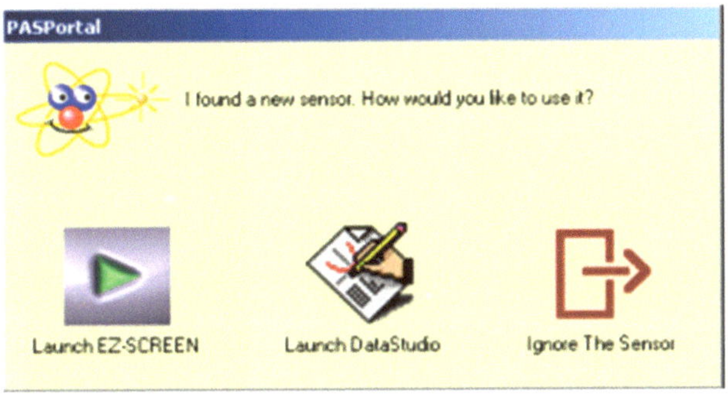

Figure 2. PASPortal window, software operation during data collection.

2.1. Sensor Specifications and Calibration

The ranges of force sensors PS2200 used in this study are 100 ± 5 N with safe overloads of up to ± 150 N. The average sampling rate in our recorded data is 20 Hz, the sensor has taken a new sample after every 0.05 s. The maximum sampling rate of sensor can be increased up to 500 Hz. The accuracy of sensor signal amplifier is $\pm$ 1 N, and a resolution of 0.003 N. We calibrated force sensors to ensure the accuracy and consistency of data recording. Calibration of force sensors were performed by hanging standard weights of 1 kg, 2 kg, 3 kg, and 4 kg on middle of handlebars of walker on right and left side. The hanging weight was distributed in rear and front sensor. By using Equations (1) and (2), the weight distributed on the rear and front sensors were summed which was approximately same to the standard weights hung on the handlebars of the walker. FL in Equation (1) shows total force on left handlebar and in Equation (2) FR shows total force on right handlebar of walker. The accuracy of the sensors was presented in Figure 3. The percentage error of the left force sensors was 1.36% and of the right force sensors were 1.18%.

$$\mathrm{FL} = \mathbf{Fs}RLs + \mathbf{Fs}FLs \tag{1}$$

$$\mathrm{FR} = \mathbf{Fs}RRs + \mathbf{Fs}FRs \tag{2}$$

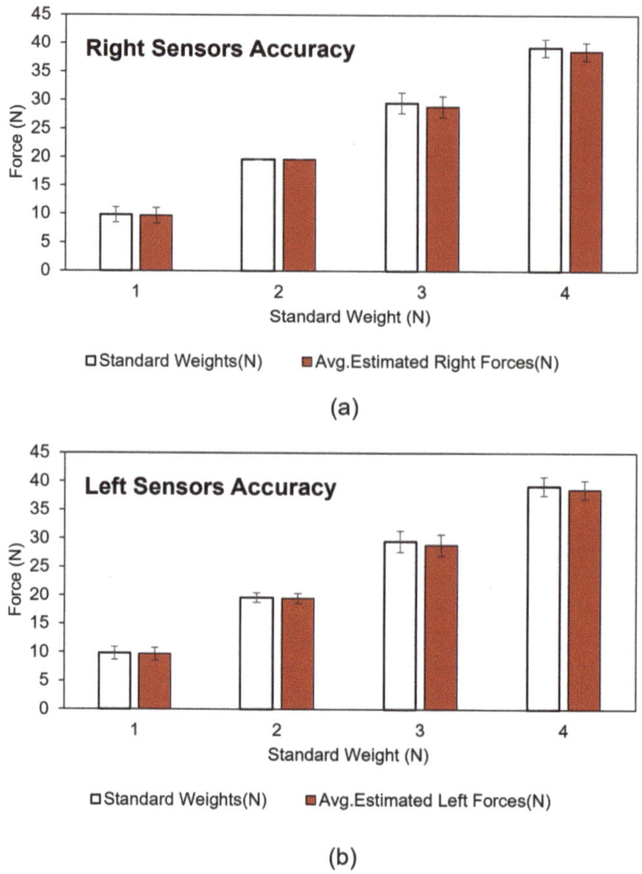

Figure 3. Validation of sensor measurement after calibration. (**a**) The sensor on the right handlebar, and (**b**) the sensor on the left handlebar.

2.2. Gait Parameters Estimation from Smart Walker with Onboard Sensors

The participant's weight distribution during walking was measured using the prototype Smart Walker. Figure 4 shows both left- and right-side forces recording from the four sensors with respect to time. Since the walker was easy to use for both groups of participants, and osteoporosis participants have experience in walker usage; thus, the data received have no significant errors and missing values. Therefore, no filters were used for data preprocessing before data analysis. The participants initiated walks by striking their right heel to the ground. At each heel strike we obtain the peak of force. The fluctuations in forces gave valuable information for the calculation of spatiotemporal gait parameters including time, stride time, stride length, cadence, step length, step time, and velocity. The force on the handlebar increased on the same side and lowered on the opposing side when users initiated a heel strike [14]. Hence, the number of steps taken by the users were easily determined by counting the number of inflection points as shown in Figure 4.

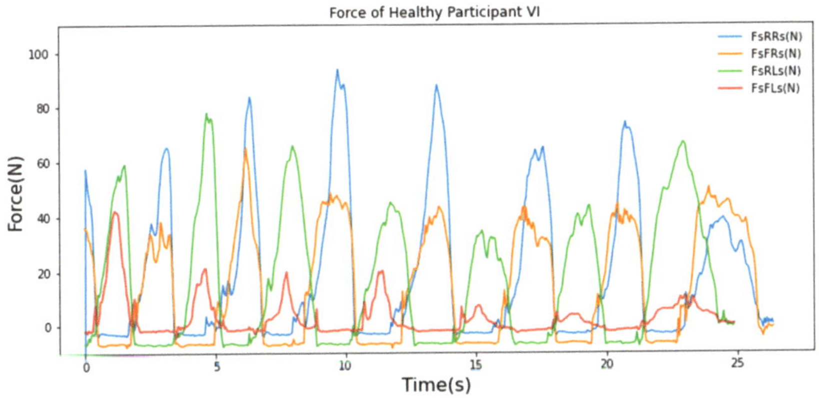

Figure 4. Force sensor reading. Force sensor on rear right side (FsRRs (N)), force sensor on rear left side (FsRLs (N)), force sensor on front right side (FsFRs (N)), and force sensor on front left side (FsFLs (N)).

For simplified data visualization, forces of two sensors attached on the left side (FsRLs + FsFLs) were added and resulted in a single force peak signal for the left heel strike, presented as the FLeft heel strike peak in Figure 5. Similarly, force measurements from the two sensors on the right side (FsRRs + FsFRs) were added to obtain one force peak signal, presented as the Fright heel strike peak in Figure 5.

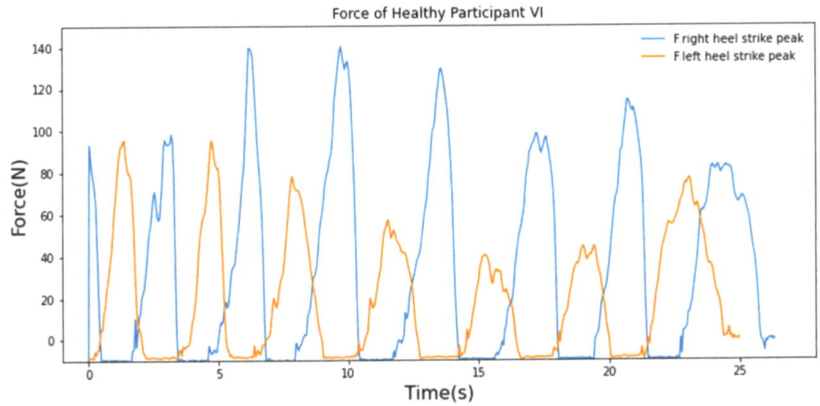

Figure 5. Sum of forces measured by sensor on rear and front (left) and on rear and front (right) during walk test using smart walker.

The differences in the forces recorded from left and right sides, occurrence of peaks at specific time and distance covered by the user, the following gait parameters were measured:

$$F_{diff} = F_{right\ heel\ strike\ peak} - F_{left\ heel\ strike\ peak} \tag{3}$$

Moreover, the following parameters were also measured:

Step Time: Average time in seconds between minimum–maximum (right) and minimum–maximum (left).

Stride Time: Average time in seconds between maximum–maximum (right) and minimum–minimum (left).

Number of steps: Number of inflection points.

Time required to complete walk: Number of seconds that a user takes to complete the walk.

Cadence: Number of steps taken * 60/time required to complete the walk.
Distance: The distance covered by user during test i.e., 10 m.
Walking Speed: Walking speed can be found by using distance (m)/time required to cover marked distance(s).
Stride length: Walking speed (m/s) * Average time in seconds between maximum–maximum (right) and minimum–minimum (left).
Step Length: walking speed (m/s) * Average time in seconds between minimum–maximum (right) and minimum–maximum (left).

$$User\ Support = F_{right\ heel\ strike\ peak} + F_{left\ heel\ strike\ peak} \quad (4)$$

After aggregating the forces exerted on the walker by the left and right sides for all walking steps, we determined the level of support provided by the user for propulsion. Equation (4) was used to calculate the amount of user support, with higher values indicating that the participant relied heavily on the walker for propulsion due to weak bone and muscle strength, resulting in high gait instability and balance issues. Conversely, lower values of user support indicated participants with better gait stability and balance who did not heavily rely on the walker for propulsion. Therefore, higher values of forces during walking were associated with gait abnormalities such as gait instability and balance issues.

2.3. Study Participants

Forty participants were recruited from The Ziauddin Hospital's Physical Therapy and Rehabilitation Centre in Karachi, Pakistan, as well as from three old age homes within Karachi, namely Anmol Zindagi, Gill Shelter Home, and Agosha-e-Afiyat. We studied 20 people with osteoporosis and 20 people without osteoporosis. In the group with osteoporosis, there were 6 males and 14 females, with a mean age of 70.85 ± 10.18 years. In the comparison group without osteoporosis, there were 11 males and 9 females with an average age of 69.85 ± 10.17 years.

The inclusion criteria for people with and without osteoporosis included being aged between 50 and 90 years old with the ability to use a walker. The group with osteoporosis included people with osteoporosis who were undergoing gait retraining using a standard walker as a rehabilitative aid and who were able to walk with a standard walker to perform their daily living activities. Exclusion criteria included individuals who had cerebral, neurological, cardiovascular or vision disorders other than osteoporosis, or individuals with osteoporosis plus othe disorders like stroke, ataxia, etc. We also excluded people who had a medical condition that affected their gait.

Ethical Approval

The Ziauddin university ethical approval policies for research conduct were followed, and informed consent was acquired from all participants.

2.4. Smart Walker Testing and Data Recording

All participants performed three walk tests at a distance of 10 m (10 m walk test) using the smart walker in the rehabilitation center, at the Ziauddin University Faculty of Physical Therapy under the supervision of a physical therapist and a nurse, as shown in Figure 6. A rehabilitation room with a plain smooth tiled floor was selected, and the volunteers were asked to walk using the smart walker on a smooth floor with shoes soaked with ink to produce marks on the floor. The participants were instructed to walk along a designated pathway while a therapist recorded the time using a stopwatch. In addition, step lengths (both right and left) and stride length were measured using a measuring tape. The walk test was used as a benchmark to validate our proposed system.

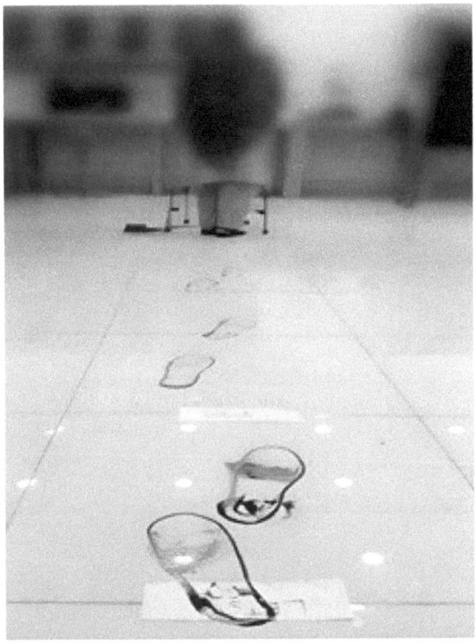

Figure 6. A 55-year-old female volunteer from the osteoporosis group performing a walk test.

3. Results

We conducted a 10 m walk test on the study participants using the smart walker to study gait patterns and associated forces exerted on the walker's handlebars during ambulation. The results showed significant differences in participants' gait dynamics. Specifically, as the participants initiated heel contact with the ground during their stride, discernible changes in the forces applied to the walker's handlebars were observed. This phenomenon was particularly evident when the participants made contact with their right heel, which correspondingly led to an augmentation in the forces registered on the right side of the walker's legs. Simultaneously, a reciprocal reduction in force was documented on the opposite side of the walker as illustrated in Figure 7.

Our analysis revealed that the inflection points in the force profiles corresponded to the instances of heel strikes during the participants' gait. This analysis allowed us to discern not only the number of heel strikes, but also the sequence in which they occurred. Evidently, the first heel strike typically originated from the right foot, marking the commencement of the gait cycle. The observation and quantification of these inflection points and heel strikes provided us with a precise and quantifiable measure of the number of steps taken by each participant during the 10 m walk test.

Figure 7 shows the generated graphs in Pasco Capstone software for the sensor recording on the walker, which measured the forces exerted by the upper limbs on the handlebars of the walker during walking. The graphical data was exported to an MS Excel file for the extraction of gait parameters. Analysis of the data revealed that users with osteoporosis exerted more force on the walker for propulsion compared to healthy users, as seen in Figure 7. Specifically, in Figure 7b, people with osteoporosis put over 100 N of body weight on the walker, while in Figure 7a, people without osteoporosis placed less than 100 N of their body weight on the walker.

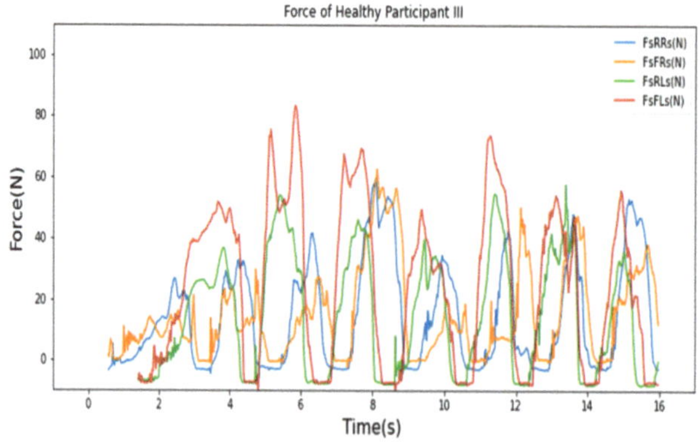

(a)

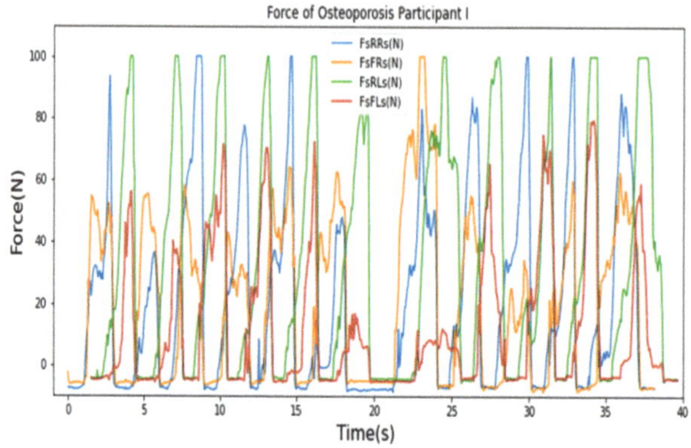

(b)

Figure 7. Force sensor readings at every heel strike during the 10 m walk test. (**a**) People without osteoporosis, (**b**) people with osteoporosis.

The one-way analysis of variance (ANOVA) or F test was performed in order to compare the two participant groups in terms of gait parameters. The results of this analysis, as well as the participants' demographic characteristics, are shown in Table 2. The results of the F test showed that the two groups were significantly different for the following four variables:

1. For average left step length, the *p*-value was 0.03, ($p(x \leq F) = 0.01$). The test statistic F was 0.350, which was not in the 95% region of acceptance: [0.3958: 2.5265]. S1/S2 = 0.59, was not in the 95% region of acceptance: [0.629: 1.589]. The 95% confidence interval of σ12/σ22 was: [0.138, 0.886].
2. The *p*-value for time was found to be 0.00, ($p(x \leq F) = 0.000$). The test statistic F was 0.186, which was not in the 95% region of acceptance: [0.395: 2.526]. S1/S2 = 0.43, was not in the 95% region of acceptance: [0.629: 1.589]. The 95% confidence interval of σ12/σ22 was: [0.073, 0.470].
3. For walking speed, the *p*-value was found to be 0.02, ($p(x \leq F) = 0.988$). The test statistic F was 2.961, which was not in the 95% region of acceptance: [0.395: 2.526. S1/S2 = 1.72, was not in the 95% region of acceptance: [0.629: 1.589]. The 95% confidence interval of σ12/σ22 was: [1.172, 7.481].
4. The *p*-value for average stride length was 0.02, ($p(x \leq F) = 0.012$). The test statistic F was 0.342, which was not in the 95% region of acceptance: [0.395: 2.526]. S1/S2 = 0.591, was not in the 95% region of acceptance: [0.629: 1.589]. The 95% confidence interval of σ12/σ22 was: [0.135, 0.865].

Table 2. Comparison of spatiotemporal parameters between participants with and without osteoporosis taken from the smart walker, after a 10 m walk test while using the smart walker prototype. Bold p-values represent significant differences.

Gait Parameters	Participants without Osteoporosis	Participants with Osteoporosis	p-Value
	Mean ± Standard Deviation	Mean ± Standard Deviation	
Age	69.85 ± 10.17	70.85 ± 10.18	
Total Distance covered (m)	10 ± 0.00	10 ± 0.00	
The number of steps counted	19.00 ± 2.83	26.4 ± 2.65	0.69
Time (s)	14.47± 3.23	33.75 ± 7.48	**0.00**
Average Left Step Length (m)	0.49 ± 0.05	0.25 ± 0.09	**0.03**
Average Right Step Length (m)	0.51 ± 0.08	0.29 ± 0.12	0.08
Average Left Step Time (s)	0.63 ± 0.13	0.90 ± 0.21	0.15
Average Right Step Time (s)	0.68 ± 0.12	0.99 ± 0.26	0.57
Walking speed (m/s)	0.72 ± 0.13	0.31 ± 0.07	**0.02**
Cadence (steps/min)	83.49 ± 15.37	47.72 ± 12.28	0.15
Average Stride Time (s)	1.35 ± 0.23	1.83± 0.23	0.56
Average Stride Length (m)	0.99 ± 0.11	0.54 ± 0.18	**0.02**

For the rest of the parameters, the two participant groups did not differ significantly ($p > 0.05$).

The results of the 10 m walk test showed that the people with osteoporosis tended to swing their leg slowly while walking, which significantly increased the time taken to take the next step. Consequently, their right and left step time, stride time, and time to complete the walk test were prolonged as shown in Figure 8. The average stride length of the people with osteoporosis decreased by 58.82% in comparison to that of people without osteoporosis while their cadence was higher compared to the people without osteoporosis, as shown in Figure 9. Moreover, People with osteoporosis walked 20.38% slower than people without osteoporosis, as can be seen in Figure 10.

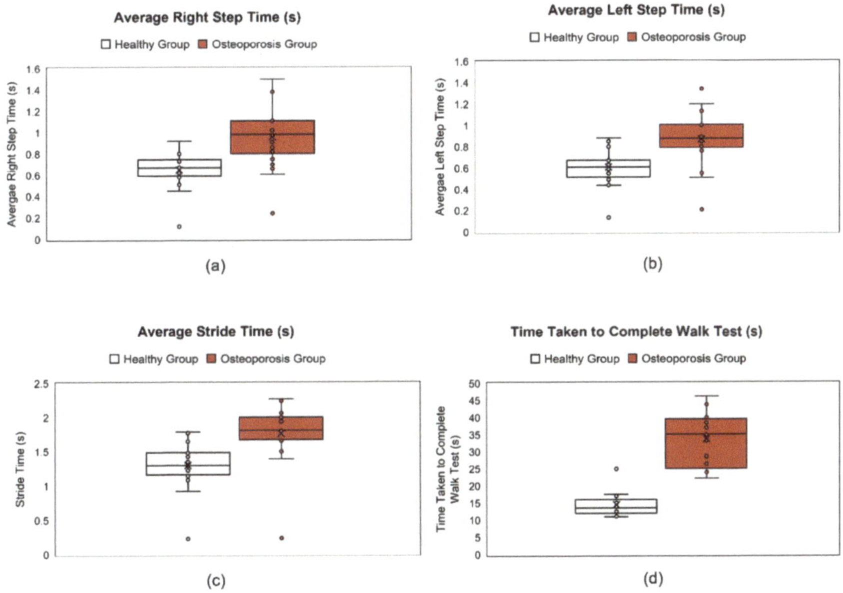

Figure 8. Graphical representation of spatiotemporal gait parameters of people with and without osteoporosis. (**a**) Average right step time, (**b**) average left step time, (**c**) stride time, and (**d**) average time taken to complete walk test.

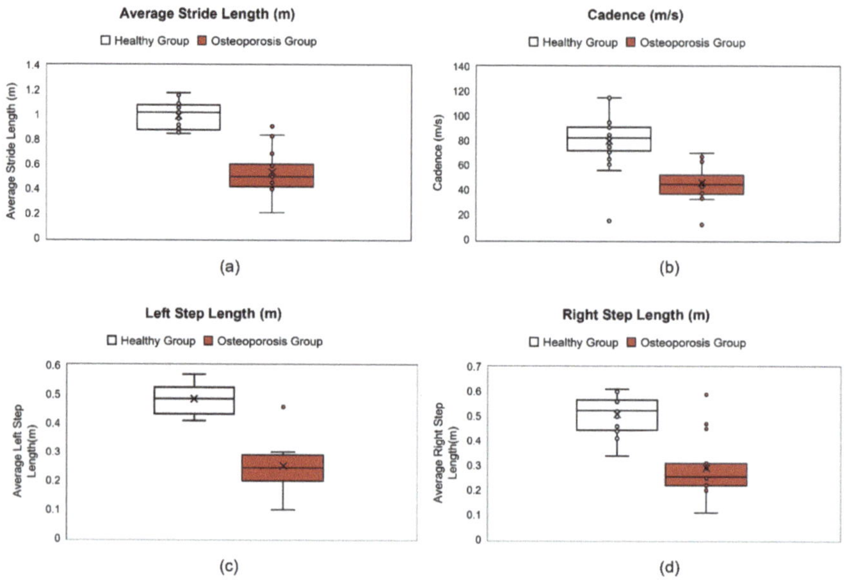

Figure 9. Graphical representation of spatiotemporal gait parameters of people with and without osteoporosis. (**a**) Average right step length, (**b**) average left step length, (**c**) average stride length, and (**d**) average cadence.

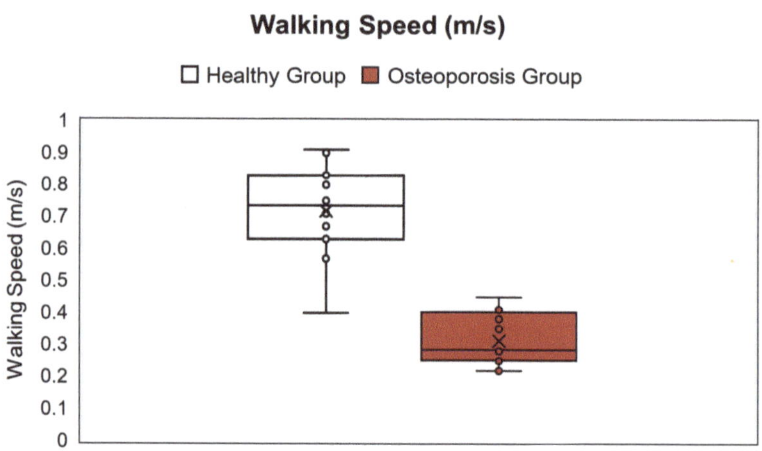

Figure 10. Average walking speed of people with and without osteoporosis.

4. Discussion

In this study, we developed and tested a smart walker prototype for monitoring gait along with providing support to users with walking disabilities. We found statistical differences in spatiotemporal gait parameters comparing people in Karachi, Pakistan, aged 50 to 90 years with and without osteoporosis. The smart walker does not need specific clothes, infrastructure, treadmills, or wearable devices. It can be used daily to assess the efficacy of therapeutic interventions provided by a physical therapist during rehabilitation process at home through self-monitoring of the number of force peaks recorded at a fixed distance. As the user's gait improves, the number of steps taken will decrease while the length of their stride will increase. The recorded data can be electronically shared with the therapist for evaluation to guide future follow-up sessions.

The gait parameters were highly affected in participants with osteoporosis compared with healthy users. It was seen that healthy adults in the age range of 50 to 90 years who do not have any significant chronic health conditions have a greater stride length, step length, cadence, and walking velocity; moreover, the stride time and average step time were lower compared with those of the osteoporotic participants because a healthy adult participant would have little or no fear of falling [35]. Thereby, people without osteoporosis took longer and a smaller number of steps to cover the 10 m marked distance compared with people with osteoporosis. The data acquired by our prototype are in accordance with the previous literature. For example, short maximal step length and slow 10 m walking speed are associated with osteoporosis in elderly women [36].

Pain due to osteoporosis may also be a factor affecting in altering spatiotemporal gait parameters. Most of our participants with osteoporosis expressed that they have trouble walking at a brisk pace and take short strides due to pain in their lower limbs while walking. Out of these patients, 16 were unable to provide us with three consecutive walk tests on the same day for the purpose of obtaining an average reading. As a result, we allocated three days to each of these patients, conducting one test per day.

A primary purpose of a standard walker is partial weight bearing of the user [37]. It was observed that the people with osteoporosis put more force on the walker while walking, in comparison to the people without osteoporosis. Since the metabolic cost of using a four-footed walker is already high [38], in the absence of any preliminary data, we cannot make a conclusive deduction. It is possible that the damage done to the bones and joints by osteoporosis increases the overall metabolic cost of walking and thus increases the force applied on our smart walker even higher [16]. Further research can explore if any correlation exists between osteoporosis and increased weight bearing.

The advantages of our proposed system include that it is portable, can be used anywhere at any time, and is economical. It has been validated with both healthy and unhealthy participants, and tests have successfully shown that the resulting gait parameters are consistent with those obtained from clinical studies. The results of our methodology are relevant to the diagnosis of people with osteoporosis by therapists. The system is easy to operate at home, allowing the user to avoid daily trips to the clinic for monitoring and enabling the recorded data to be saved according to date. By daily monitoring of the user's gait parameters, a clinician can assess the effectiveness of recommended treatment plans on a daily and weekly basis and make informed decisions about the best course of treatment for people with osteoporosis.

Usually, instrumented gait analysis via smart assistive devices is more economical in comparison to the conventional method of motion capture. Even these devices have a starting range of USD 6000 [39]. Our proposed system costs only USD 1000, making it more affordable for people in general, and for people in developing countries in particular. In addition to being cost-effective, our proposed system also offers a user-friendly interface and easy setup, eliminating the need for specialized training or technical expertise. This makes it accessible to a wider range of users, including those with limited resources or knowledge in gait analysis.

Smart Walker did not take into account how confounding variables given by various other factors might affect the gait; it is expected that in a clinical setting, people with osteoporosis also have comorbidities that impact the gait, some of them being quite common, such as joint pain, sores on feet, calluses, ingrown toenails, inner ear issues, poor lower limb circulation, poor vision, etc., whereas others are more serious, such as arthritis, herniated disk, or stroke [40]. The smart walker is wired, and users need to use the device at a fixed distance during gait monitoring; there is no direct transmission of data from walker to clinicians. This is rather a technical limitation that we considered acceptable in our prototype which focused on collecting data and identifying gait patterns related to osteoporosis. Future wireless prototypes with the ability to transmit data to the clinician will add to the functionality of the smart walker.

Further research is needed to analyze how other conditions might affect the accuracy of our proposed method and to determine if the smart walker may be useful in evaluating these conditions as risk factors for gait impairment.

5. Conclusions

The gait of people with osteoporosis observed via the proposed non-wheeled smart walker differed from that of people without osteoporosis, in terms of walking step length, stride length and the time taken to complete the 10 m walk test. The smart walker was successful in capturing gait characteristics in real-time, without the hassle of any wearable sensors or motion capture. Additional investigation is required to ascertain whether the smart walker could be a practical tool in assessing these conditions as risk factors for gait impairment and to examine how other conditions might impact the accuracy of our proposed method.

6. Patents

We filed a patent for a smart walker for lower limb disabilities at the international property organization of Pakistan (IPO).

Author Contributions: Conceptualization, N.E., S.J.K., S.-D.S. and F.A.; methodology, N.E., S.J.K., M.F. and E.T.; software, N.E., A.I.-A.-D., A.P., F.A. and S.J.K.; validation, E.T., A.I.-A.-D., A.P. and F.A., formal analysis, N.E., S.J.K., F.A. and M.F.; investigation, N.E., S.J.K. and F.A.; resources, S.J.K., F.A., M.F. and N.E.; data curation, N.E., S.J.K., A.P. and A.I.-A.-D.; writing—original draft preparation, N.E.; writing—review and editing, S.-D.S., A.I.-A.-D. and F.A.; visualization, S.J.K., M.F. and N.E.; supervision, S.J.K. and F.A.; project administration, N.E., S.J.K. and F.A.; funding acquisition, S.-D.S., E.T., A.P. and A.I.-A.-D. All authors have read and agreed to the published version of the manuscript.

Funding: This research received no external funding.

Institutional Review Board Statement: The study was conducted in accordance with the Declaration of Helsinki, and approved by the Institutional Review Board (or Ethics Committee) of Ziauddin University (protocol code ERC/ZUFESTM/002 and date of approval is June 2023) for studies involving humans.

Informed Consent Statement: Informed consent was obtained from all subjects involved in the study.

Data Availability Statement: The data presented in this study are available on request from the corresponding authors. The dataset is not publicly available due to ethical privacy of participants involved in this study.

Conflicts of Interest: The authors declare no conflict of interest.

References

1. Waters, D.; Hale, L.; Grant, A.; Herbison, P.; Goulding, A.J. Osteoporosis and gait and balance disturbances in older sarcopeni obese New Zealanders. *Osteoporos. Int.* **2010**, *21*, 351–357. [CrossRef] [PubMed]
2. Weinhandl, J.T.; Irmischer, B.S.; Sievert, Z.A.J.A.B. Effects of gait speed of femoroacetabular joint forces. *Appl. Bionics Biomech* **2017**, *2017*, 6432969. [CrossRef] [PubMed]
3. Löfgren, N.; Halvarsson, A.; Ståhle, A.; Franzén, E. Gait characteristics in older women with osteoporosis and fear of falling. *Eur J. Physiother.* **2013**, *15*, 139–145. [CrossRef]
4. Aveiro, M.; Granito, R.; Navega, M.; Driusso, P.; Oishi, J. Influence of a physical training program on muscle strength, balance and gait velocity among women with osteoporosis. *Braz. J. Phys. Ther.* **2006**, *10*, 441–448. [CrossRef]
5. Rathinam, C.; Bateman, A.; Peirson, J.; Skinner, J.J.G. Observational gait assessment tools in paediatrics—A systematic review *Gait Posture* **2014**, *40*, 279–285. [CrossRef] [PubMed]
6. Marin, J.; Marin, J.J.; Blanco, T.; de la Torre, J.; Salcedo, I.; Martitegui, E.J.A.S. Is my patient improving? Individualized gait analysis in rehabilitation. *Appl. Sci.* **2020**, *10*, 8558. [CrossRef]
7. Chan, S.C.; Chan, Y.T.n.; Chong, Y.Z. A low-cost human gait analysis system. In Proceedings of the Kuala Lumpur International Conference on Biomedical Engineering, Kuala Lumpur, Malaysia, 28 July 2021; pp. 197–203.
8. Zhang, P.; Zhang, Y. Video methods for gait analysis in daily environment. In Proceedings of the 13th International Conference on Signal Processing Systems (ICSPS 2021), Shanghai, China, 12–15 November 2021; pp. 374–380.
9. Felius, R.A.; Geerars, M.; Bruijn, S.M.; van Dieën, J.H.; Wouda, N.C.; Punt, M.J.S. Reliability of IMU-based gait assessment in clinical stroke rehabilitation. *Sensors* **2022**, *22*, 908. [CrossRef] [PubMed]

10. Mohan, D.M.; Khandoker, A.H.; Wasti, S.A.; Ismail Ibrahim Ismail Alali, S.; Jelinek, H.F.; Khalaf, K. Assessment methods of post-stroke gait: A scoping review of technology-driven approaches to gait characterization and analysis. *Front. Neurol.* **2021**, *12*, 650024. [CrossRef]
11. Farid, L.; Jacobs, D.; Do Santos, J.; Simon, O.; Gracies, J.-M.; Hutin, E. FeetMe® Monitor-connected insoles are a valid and reliable alternative for the evaluation of gait speed after stroke. *Top. Stroke Rehabil.* **2021**, *28*, 127–134. [CrossRef]
12. Park, S.J.; Hussain, I.; Hong, S.; Kim, D.; Park, H.; Benjamin, H.C.M. Real-time gait monitoring system for consumer stroke prediction service. In Proceedings of the IEEE International Conference on Consumer Electronics (ICCE), Las Vegas, NV, USA, 4–6 January 2020; pp. 1–4.
13. Atia, C.O.; Ojeda, M.; Béjar, J.; Martínez, A.B. An pproach to Gait Analysis from Human-Rollator Interaction: The i-Walker. *Artif. Intell. Res. Dev. Curr. Chall. New Trends Appl.* **2018**, *308*, 335.
14. Ballesteros, J.; Urdiales, C.; Martinez, A.B.; Tirado, M. Gait analysis for challenged users based on a rollator equipped with force sensors. In Proceedings of the IEEE/RSJ International Conference on Intelligent Robots and Systems (IROS), Hamburg, Germany, 28 September–2 October 2015; pp. 5587–5592.
15. Ballesteros, J.; Urdiales, C.; Martinez, A.B.; Tirado, M. Automatic Assessment of a Rollator-User's Condition During Rehabilitation Using the i-Walker Platform. *IEEE Trans. Neural Syst. Rehabil. Eng.* **2017**, *25*, 2009–2017. [CrossRef] [PubMed]
16. Ballesteros, J.; Tudela, A.; Caro-Romero, J.R.; Urdiales, C. Weight-Bearing Estimation for Cane Users by Using Onboard Sensors. *Sensors* **2019**, *19*, 509. [CrossRef] [PubMed]
17. Caro-Romero, J.R.; Ballesteros, J.; Garcia-Lagos, F.; Urdiales, C.; Sandoval, F. A Neural Network for Stance Phase detection in smart cane users. In Proceedings of the Advances in Computational Intelligence: 15th International Work-Conference on Artificial Neural Networks, IWANN 2019, Gran Canaria, Spain, 12–14 June 2019; pp. 310–321.
18. Ballesteros, J.; Urdiales, C.; Martinez, A.B.; Van Dieën, J.H.J.S. On gait analysis estimation errors using force sensors on a smart rollator. *Sensors* **2016**, *16*, 1896. [CrossRef] [PubMed]
19. Papageorgiou, X.S.; Chalvatzaki, G.; Tzafestas, C.S.; Maragos, P. Hidden Markov modeling of human normal gait using laser range finder for a mobility assistance robot. In Proceedings of the IEEE International Conference on Robotics and Automation (ICRA), Hong Kong, China, 31 May–7 June 2014; pp. 482–487.
20. Fujimoto, A.; Matsumoto, N.; Jiang, Y.; Togo, S.; Teshigawara, S.; Yokoi, H. Gait analysis based speed control of walking assistive robot. In Proceedings of the IEEE International Conference on Intelligence and Safety for Robotics (ISR), Shenyang, China, 24–27 August 2018; pp. 88–92.
21. Palermo, M.; Lopes, J.M.; André, J.; Matias, A.C.; Cerqueira, J.; Santos, C.P. A multi-camera and multimodal dataset for posture and gait analysis. *Sci. Data* **2022**, *9*, 603. [CrossRef] [PubMed]
22. Yan, Q.; Huang, J.; Wu, D.; Yang, Z.; Wang, Y.; Hasegawa, Y.; Fukuda, T. Intelligent Gait Analysis and Evaluation System Based on Cane Robot. *IEEE Trans. Neural Syst. Rehabil. Eng.* **2022**, *30*, 2916–2926. [CrossRef] [PubMed]
23. Page, S.; Martins, M.M.; Saint-Bauzel, L.; Santos, C.P.; Pasqui, V. Fast embedded feet pose estimation based on a depth camera for smart walker. In Proceedings of the IEEE International Conference on Robotics and Automation (ICRA), Seattle, WA, USA, 26–30 May 2015; pp. 4224–4229.
24. Postolache, O.; Pereira, J.D.; Viegas, V.; Girão, P.S. Gait rehabilitation assessment based on microwave Doppler radars embedded in walkers. In Proceedings of the IEEE International Symposium on Medical Measurements and Applications (MeMeA) Proceedings, Turin, Italy, 7–9 May 2015; pp. 208–213.
25. Ojeda, M.; Cortés, A.; Béjar, J.; Cortés, U. Automatic classification of gait patterns using a smart rollator and the BOSS model. In Proceedings of the 11th PErvasive Technologies Related to Assistive Environments Conference, Corfu, Greece, 26–29 June 2018; pp. 384–390.
26. Werner, C.; Chalvatzaki, G.; Papageorgiou, X.S.; Tzafestas, C.S.; Bauer, J.M.; Hauer, K. Assessing the concurrent validity of a gait analysis system integrated into a smart walker in older adults with gait impairments. *Clin. Rehabil.* **2019**, *33*, 1682–1687. [CrossRef] [PubMed]
27. Fernandez-Carmona, M.; Ballesteros, J.; Díaz-Boladeras, M.; Parra-Llanas, X.; Urdiales, C.; Gómez-De-Gabriel, J.M. Walk-IT: An Open-Source Modular Low-Cost Smart Rollator. *Sensors* **2022**, *22*, 2086. [CrossRef] [PubMed]
28. Viegas, V.; Pereira, J.M.D.; Postolache, O.; Girão, P.S. Monitoring Walker Assistive Devices: A Novel Approach Based on Load Cells and Optical Distance Measurements. *Sensors* **2018**, *18*, 540. [CrossRef]
29. Cimolin, V.; Galli, M. Summary measures for clinical gait analysis: A literature review. *Gait Posture* **2014**, *39*, 1005–1010. [CrossRef]
30. Zijlstra, W.; Hof, A.L. Assessment of spatio-temporal gait parameters from trunk accelerations during human walking. *Gait Posture* **2003**, *18*, 1–10. [CrossRef]
31. Lee, G.; Ohnuma, T.; Chong, N.Y. Design and control of JAIST active robotic walker. *Intell. Serv. Robot.* **2010**, *3*, 125–135. [CrossRef]
32. Morone, G.; Annicchiarico, R.; Iosa, M.; Federici, A.; Paolucci, S.; Cortés, U.; Caltagirone, C. Overground walking training with the i-Walker, a robotic servo-assistive device, enhances balance in patients with subacute stroke: A randomized controlled trial. *J. Neuroeng.Rehabil.* **2016**, *13*. [CrossRef] [PubMed]
33. Andreetto, M.; Divan, S.; Fontanelli, D.; Palopoli, L. Passive robotic walker path following with bang-bang hybrid control paradigm. In Proceedings of the IEEE/RSJ International Conference on Intelligent Robots and Systems (IROS), Daejeon, Republic of Korea, 9–14 October 2016; pp. 1054–1060.

34. Mehr, J.K.; Akbari, M.; Faridi, P.; Xing, H.; Mushahwar, V.K.; Tavakoli, M. Artificial-Intelligence-Powered Lower Limb Assistive Devices: Future of Home Care Technologies. *Adv. Intell. Syst.* **2023**, *5*, 2200361. [CrossRef]
35. Hamed, K.; Roaldsen, K.; Halvarsson, A.J.O.i. Fear of falling serves as protection and signifies potential danger: A qualitative study to conceptualise the phrase "fear of falling" in women with osteoporosis. *Osteoporos. Int.* **2021**, *32*, 2563–2570. [CrossRef]
36. Park, H.; Park, S.; Komatsu, T.; Kaminai, T.; Mutoh, Y. Walking Characteristics and Bone Mineral Density in Community-dwelling Elderly Women: A Cross-Sectional Study. *Phys. Educ. Med. Res.* **2003**, *4*, 11–19.
37. Lopes, S.; Filipe, L.; Silva, R.; Cruz, A.; Parreira, P.; Couto, F.; Bernardes, R.; Apóstolo, J.; Roseiro, L.; Malça, C. An Innovative Concept for a Walker with a Self-Locking Mechanism Using a Single Mechanical Approach. *Int. J. Environ. Res. Public Heal.* **2019**, *16*, 1671. [CrossRef] [PubMed]
38. Priebe, J.R.; Kram, R. Why is walker-assisted gait metabolically expensive? *Gait Posture* **2011**, *34*, 265–269. [CrossRef] [PubMed]
39. Mann, W.C. *Smart Technology for Aging, Disability, and Independence: The State of the Science*; John Wiley & Sons: Hoboken, NJ, USA, 2005
40. Puth, M.-T.; Klaschik, M.; Schmid, M.; Weckbecker, K.; Münster, E. Prevalence and comorbidity of osteoporosis—A cross-sectional analysis on 10,660 adults aged 50 years and older in Germany. *BMC Musculoskelet. Disord.* **2018**, *19*, 144. [CrossRef]

applied sciences

MDPI

Article

The Design and Testing of an Additive Manufacturing-Obtained Compliant Mechanism for the Complex Personalisation of Lenses in Clinical Optometry

Victor Constantin, Daniel Comeagă, Bogdan Grămescu *, Daniel Besnea and Edgar Moraru

Department of Mechatronics and Precision Mechanics, Faculty of Mechanical Engineering and Mechatronics, National University of Science and Technology POLITEHNICA Bucharest, 060042 Bucharest, Romania
* Correspondence: bogdan.gramescu@upb.ro

Abstract: The precision needed in optometric measurements for the correct customization of progressive lenses usually falls short of what is required for accurate prescriptions. This usually stems from the fact that most measurements are obtained using outdated methods, employing either rulers or protractors. While there is equipment available for precise measurements, the cost of purchase and ownership is usually prohibitive. In this context, due to constant progress in high-resolution cameras along with the processing power of handheld devices, another solution has presented itself in different iterations in the past decade, as put forward by different manufacturers of optical lenses. Such a system comprises a mobile computing device with image capture and processing capabilities (tablet or smartphone), along with a marker support system to be mounted on the user's glasses frames. Aside from cost, the ease of implementation and usage, the advantage of such a system is that the parameters, as measured, allow for better customization, since the eyewear is already in the position in which it will be used. It allows the optometrist to measure parameters such as interpupillary distance, pantoscopic angle and the curvature of the eyewear in relation to the user's own specific shape and size. This paper proposes a model of a marker support system that is easy to use, precise, low in cost and has minimal impact on the measurements obtained by the optometrist. As such, this paper examines the steps for determining the shape needed for supports in relation to the measurements that need to be taken; a finite element analysis of the support was proposed, along with various tests and modifications that were made to the device until a specific shape and material combination was found that satisfied all of the parameters required. An experimental model of the system was produced and tested on a wide variety of glasses frames with good results, as presented in the following work.

Keywords: compliant mechanism; optometry; progressive lens customisation; additive manufacturing

1. Introduction

A model for a compliant mechanism to be used in the structure of a marker support system was developed and tested by various methods [1], with a final result being obtained in the form of the shape in Figure 1. The model took into account a force of 35 N maximum to be applied to each side of the marker support system, with PLA being used as a material to build the part by using Fusion Deposition Methods—thus obtaining a total stroke of approximately 30 mm, allowing for eyewear with a total height of up to 60 mm to be measured.

The first applications of additive manufacturing (AM) technologies in medicine date back to the end of the 20th century and refer to achievements in dental prosthetics and implantology [2,3]. Since then, these manufacturing methods have greatly developed, have exponentially progressed and are applied in almost all branches of the medical field, opening new horizons for mankind and improving the quality of life [4]. Nowadays, there are many uses of 3D printing for various complex prosthetic constructions applied in the dental field, or other types of orthopaedic prostheses [5–7], and these uses include making models and prototypes for educational purposes [8], preparing/planning operations [9], creating surgical instruments [10] and other personalized medical tools that are anatomically suitable for each patient, applications in the field of pharmacology research [11] and even the creation of living tissues or cells [12].

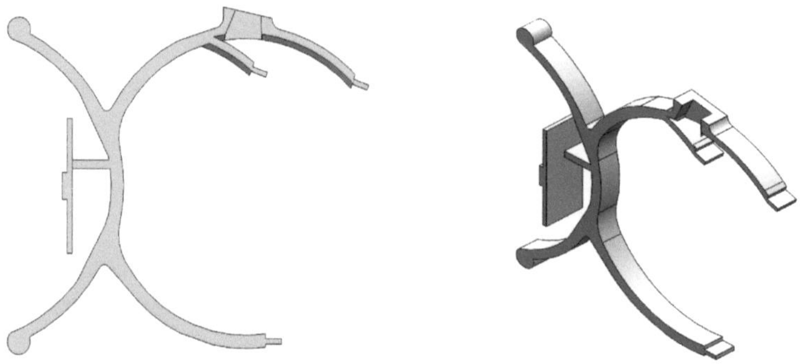

Figure 1. Front and isometric views of the model used for lateral marker support.

There have been recent evolutions in the optical and optometric fields, and the new applications of additive technologies have been felt [13,14]. For example, the appearance of personalized glasses frames obtained using additive technologies [15] can be considered a beginning for the further development and revolutionizing of the optometric field, respecting all the physiological and anatomical features of a person and taking into account the client's desires and his anthropometric data. Selective laser deposition technology [16,17] using metal/polymeric powders has proven to be the most suitable for the manufacturing of frames, and its advantage is the almost complete absence of scraps, unlike traditional production where considerable material losses are recorded. Additive technologies can also allow for the production of various lenses [18] and innovative and multifunctional components, which can simplify, optimize and miniaturize optical systems, being able to perfect medical instruments, equipment for scientific research or household equipment. It is also worth mentioning the efforts and special progress made in the ophthalmological field, using bioprinting for corneal reconstruction and regeneration or the creation of other eye tissues such as retina or conjunctiva [19–21]. Such research is in the advanced testing/research phase and has great prospects for use in the field in the future, bringing important contributions to the development of this medical area and major benefits for people with ocular disabilities.

Therefore, surely 3D printing will radically change the activity of an ophthalmologist, optician or optometrist for the better. The application described in this paper can fall into the category of assistive systems for optometric applications, and, as a basis for realization, utilized thermoplastic extrusion technology—FDM (fused deposition modelling) [1,22].

This paper demonstrates the steps that were taken in the design, preliminary finite element analysis, fabrication and testing of a novel shape and model of a marker support system for evaluating the measurements needed for obtaining specific parameters in the customisation of progressive lenses. The model was designed using flexible parts that would allow the position of markers mounted on the system to be influenced by specific parameters in a glasses' frame, as well as the relative position of the frame to the patient. The marker support system was 3D modelled and simulated with good results, which prompted the manufacturing of the system using FDM technology. Following initial tests, the support system was employed to test for specific parameters with good results in simple, preliminary trials.

2. Complete System Description

Shapes and materials previously studied [1] were used to create and assemble the system as presented in Figure 2a,b. The first of the two shows a frontal view of the marker support system, as viewed by the optometrist. It comprises two compliant mechanisms: (1), one for each of the two openings of the glasses frames on which the system will sit by means of supports (2), (3) and (4). A large number of supports is needed to accommodate a large number of the shapes and sizes of glasses frames. As such, the mounting of the device onto a pair of glasses is performed by applying a force of up to 30 N to each side of the frame using handles (8), resulting in a larger opening between supports (2) and (4), as well as (2) and (3). Next, supports (3) and (4) are placed on the upper side of the frame, (2) is placed on the lower side and the force is removed. The bridge between the two lateral compliant mechanisms is flexible, allowing the support to match the glasses frame's curvature. The bridge comprises a central fixed section (6), a flexible portion (5) and a fixed marker support section (7). Lateral marker support is offered by means of support (9).

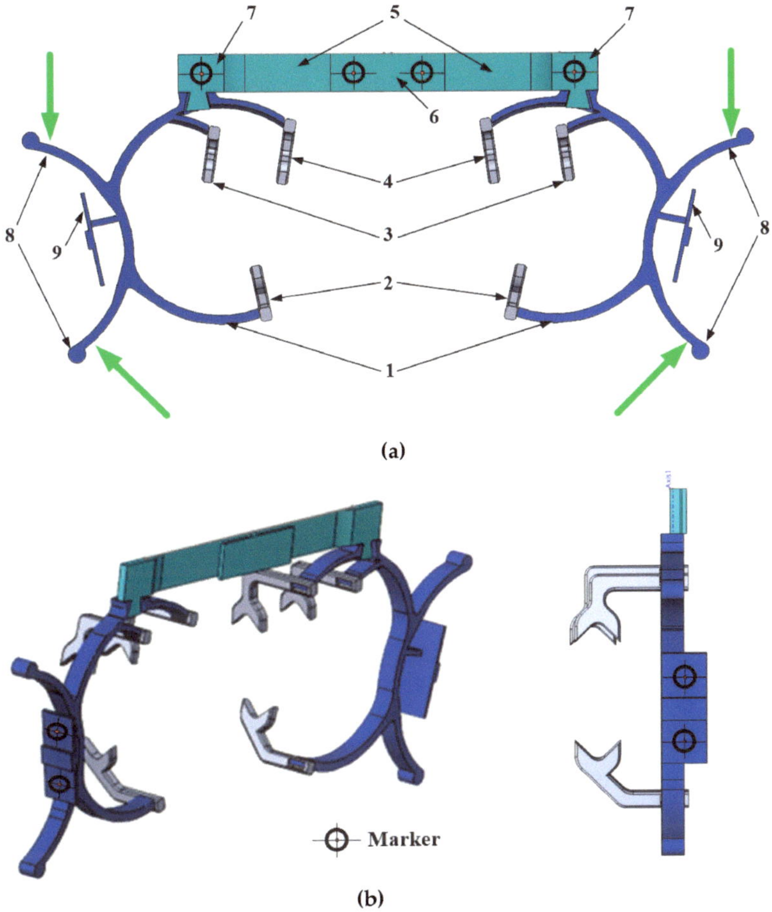

Figure 2. Views of the complete optometric model used for lateral marker support: (**a**)—front view; (**b**)—isometric and lateral views.

The device is built in modules to both allow, in some instances, for different materials to be used and improve on some of the parameters of the final product. Printing three separate parts allows for better quality, lower print times and a wider range of desktop printers that might be used to manufacture the device.

Regarding the movement of the markers due to the deformation of the device, both the lateral (side) markers and the central ones are mounted on small, single cantilever plates that are not deformed during the mounting process. The distance between these points is known (calibrated) and serves as a reference during the measurements. The idea of directly printing the colour markers was certainly considered; issues with material colour consistency convinced us to use conventionally printed colour markers.

The support is used to position a set of markers relative to a user's face and determine, using a method to be discussed in another paper, dimensions specific to the user's facial parameters and chosen glasses frames. It allows for the acquisition of parameters such as the following: pupillary and interpupillary distance, curvature of the glasses frames, pantoscopic angle on both sides of the user's face as well as measurements related to customizing the lens to the glasses frames. The markers used are manufactured on adhesive, low-gloss paper of a specific colour and are positioned using a specially made stencil in order to guarantee their position. Figure 3 shows a chart of the measurements that can be taken using this system. This system allows all necessary parameters to be determined by taking both a close-up and a far picture of the patient wearing the glasses and marker support assembly.

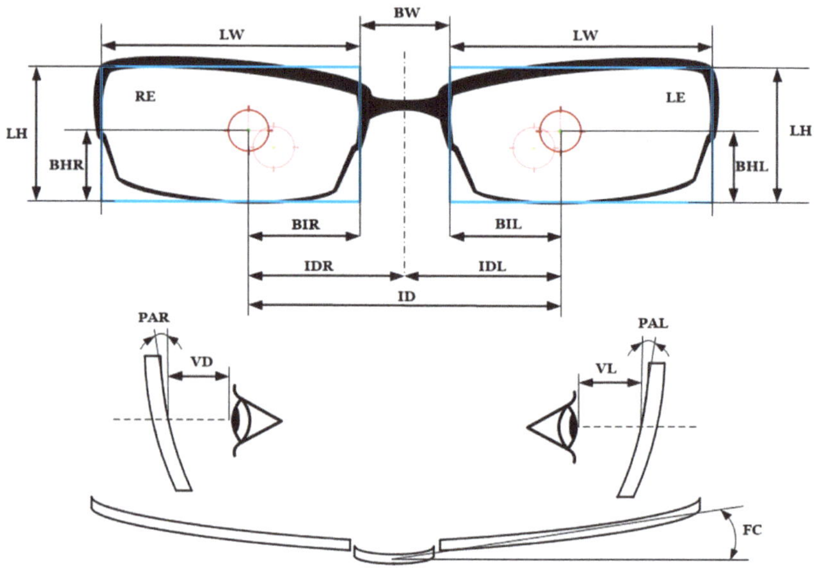

Figure 3. Measurements taken by the system.

Among the measurements that can be taken are the following: IDR (interpupillary distance, total as well as right IDR and left IDL), LW (lens width, both left and right), LH (lens height, left and right), BW (Bridge Width), BHR and BHL (pupil distance to lower part of lens) as well as BIL and BIR (pupil distance to lower part of lens). Along these, measurements related to vertex distance (VL and VD), distance between the pupil and lens, PAR and PAL (left and right pantoscopic angle) as well as the glasses frame curvature FC are included.

3. General Estimation of the Assembly's Mechanical Behaviour before Manufacturing

This chapter is centred on analysing the mechanical behaviour of the proposed structure, using specific numerical engineering simulation tools and the finite element method [1,23]. Currently, finite element simulations are powerful analysis instruments that have a deep theoretical basis in the solving of a wide range of technical problems [24–33], not least in the biomedical field [34,35] and including the ophthalmology/optometric field [1,36], to improve medical devices before their realization. Considering the nature of the physical and mechanical properties of the thermoplastic materials used for the FDM process, but also due to the specific peculiarities of the layered structure that make it difficult to establish a simulated numerical solution as close to reality as possible, the aim of this study is to approximate the behaviour of the structure, according to applied loads during operation, on a given type of glasses before the manufacturing of the system and to obtain preliminary results and an estimate of the displacement of the marker support system. For this purpose, a structural static type of analysis was used, and polylactic acid (PLA) was chosen as the base material in the simulation—the properties attributed to the material being the same as in the previous authors' paper [1]—with Young's modulus established experimentally [37,38].

The following paragraphs will present the stages and results obtained from the simulation of the structure of the complete compliant mechanism proposed, using the FEA method, as well as the mechanical loads that occur during its operation, using the Solid Works program. The following classical steps regarding FEA simulation were applied: designing and modelling the structure, creating the mathematical model and physical conditions—choosing the multiphysics module, assigning the material, establishing fixed geometries, assigning the loads, dividing the loads into finite elements and running and interpreting the results.

The central element of the bridge was established as fixed geometry, and mechanical loads were established as input data; a normal force of 15 N was applied to the four faces of the grasping structure, according to the loads proposed from a previous paper [1]. Additionally, torques of the absolute value of 0.002 N·m, with opposite signs around an imaginary vertical axis on the lateral faces of the bridge, were applied.

Figure 4 presents the results obtained from the FEA simulation of the complete structure proposed for the optometric application, regarding the resultant displacement on all three axes and equivalent von Mises stress. It is possible to observe how the highest values intervene in the inferior area of the grasping elements with the maximum resultant displacement value of 39.39 mm. Regarding the equivalent von Mises stresses, the most affected regions appear at the flexible part of the bridge but also appear in some areas of the grasping element, with all values nevertheless being below the yield strength of the material for the loads applied, validating the model proposed.

In Figure 5a, it is possible to notice the displacements obtained on the vertical axis (Z), i.e., the maximum openings of the mechanism resulting from the loads applied. These are values of interest, because they indicate the size of the eyeglasses on which the mechanism can operate. For example, the maximum and minimum values can be identified on the figure, i.e., the maximum displacements from the initial position of hypothetical contact surfaces with eyeglasses (11.653 mm and −1.387 mm, respectively). Summing up their absolute values, an opening of 13.04 mm can be obtained from the initial distance between the grasping elements (namely contact surfaces with eyeglasses); therefore, in the case of simulation with the proposed material and applied loads mentioned above, this mechanism is able to operate on eyeglasses with a size greater than 13 mm, compared to the initial design distance of the grasping elements of the compliant mechanism (falls within the range of eyeglasses size with which the proposed mechanism can operate). In Figure 5b, some details regarding the results of the displacement on the Y axis can be identified, following the torque applied in the area of the lateral part of the bridge, where maximum values of over 10 mm are obtained. Figure 5c illustrates the results of the movement on the Z-axis—only for the grasping elements where the maximum values, minimum values and distribution of displacements can only be seen in the mentioned areas of interest. In all of the cases in Figure 5, the initial positions of the entities of the structure are highlighted.

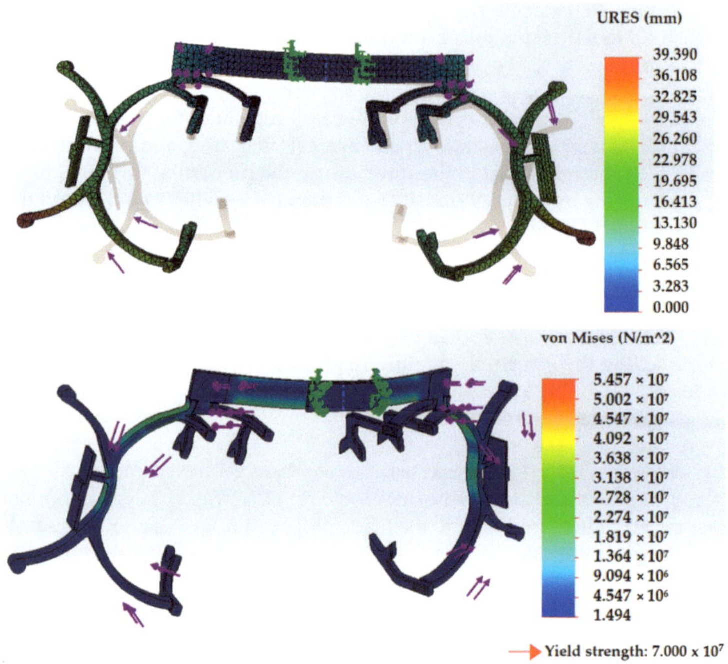

Figure 4. Obtained displacements (resultant displacement) and von Mises stress results for the compliant mechanism.

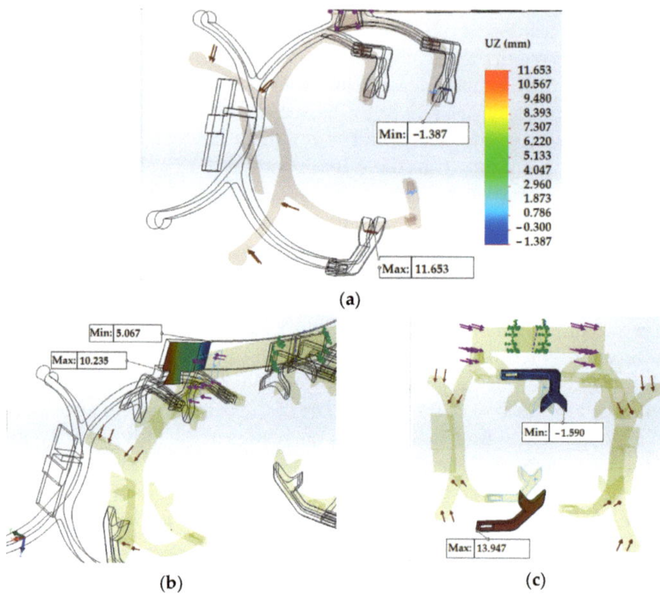

Figure 5. Some details of the results obtained after a FEA estimation of the structure proposed: (**a**)—Resulting opening of the mechanism (vertical Z axis) at 13.04 mm after load application; (**b**)—Y axis displacement of the lateral part of the bridge; (**c**)—Z axis displacement of the grasping elements.

Figure 6 presents an image depicting the simulation of the compliant mechanism's operation; in this, it is possible to observe the grasping of a certain type of eyeglasses, thereby validating the complete system model of the compliant mechanism proposed and being able to proceed with its realization and testing.

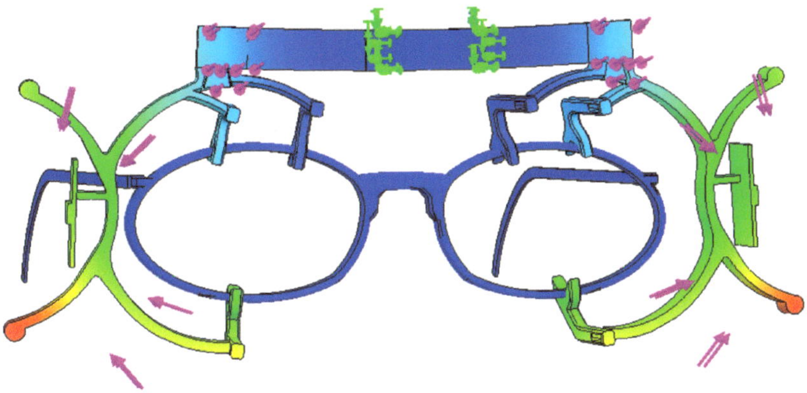

Figure 6. A simulation of the operation of the compliant mechanism proposed for the optometric field.

4. Manufacturing of a Prototype and Preliminary System Testing

Current additive manufacturing technologies allow for complex mechanisms to be tested before mass production—however, in some instances, they even allow for direct-to-customer-use manufacturing. For our designed mechanism, such a path was chosen, in that small batches could be produced and modified for specific needs in terms of the shapes of glasses frames. It is also important to note here that the current wide array of both materials, as well as composites, allow for the mechanism to be customized even further in terms of mechanical properties, look and feel, while taking into consideration that almost all of the changes to the material will, in some capacity, modify the way the mechanism transmits force and motion through elastic body transformation.

To this end, several materials were considered, of course, principally taking into consideration the notion that they should be inherently chemically inert to external use with the person wearing the glasses and the support system. Using this as a starting point and after some tests and consideration, as presented in a previous study [1], a specific version of thermoplastic polyurethane was chosen [1], with some of the material's properties being density 1.18 g/cm^3, a Young modulus of 0.396 GPa and a yield strength of 65.85 MPa. While these parameters are specific to this material and do allow for the imposed travel of the mechanism's supports at approximately 30 mm at a 35 N-applied force on each end, further research has proven that such mechanical behaviour can also be obtained by using other materials, such as specific variants of Polylactic acid PLA. Also, some studies could be performed in order to determine to what extent, for this specific shape and purpose, slicing and FDM [37–42] parameters influence compliant behaviour, as well as long term use of the system.

Regarding FDM parameters, while a general-purpose FDM slicing software was used, specific parameters were tested in order to allow for the best results, both cosmetic and structural. Regarding the actual additive manufacturing system, a general-purpose desktop cartesian system was used, Prusa i3 model, capable of temperatures that are compatible with working with materials such as TPU or Nylon. It should be noted here that, since the material is flexible, a direct drive extruder is needed, with adjustments made to the pretensioning mechanism, specific to the elasticity of the material used. As for some of the specific parameters used during slicing, a low speed was selected (20 mm/s) for the infill, with an even lower speed of 15 mm/s for the outer walls. Infill was selected as full (100%), with a wall thickness of 0.8 mm, with bottom and top walls at a minim of 1.2 mm. During several tests performed, it was concluded that, in order to obtain the best results in both elasticity and overall mechanism usability, an infill of 100% should be used. There was also no advantage to be had by experimenting with other infill percentages since, with these current parameters, all of the requirements, such as shape and weight, were met.

The physical model was tested on a wide array of shapes of glasses, with a height from approximately 27 mm up to 60 mm, with good results in terms of both ease in fixing the support and maintaining its position in use. The model was proven to allow for accurate measurements of previously specified parameters (see Figure 3). Also, the model proved to allow for movement on behalf of the patient, without disturbing the position of the device once it was fixed to the frames.

During the tests, it was determined that, while certain rarer models of frames might pose an issue—such as extremely large or small models, as the ones encountered in use for children—the model could be easily modified to fit such situations. In some cases, this can be done by simply removing the supports used to fix the device to the frames. Figure 7a–c shows the support mounted on different shapes of glasses, as empirically determined to be among the most chosen by users.

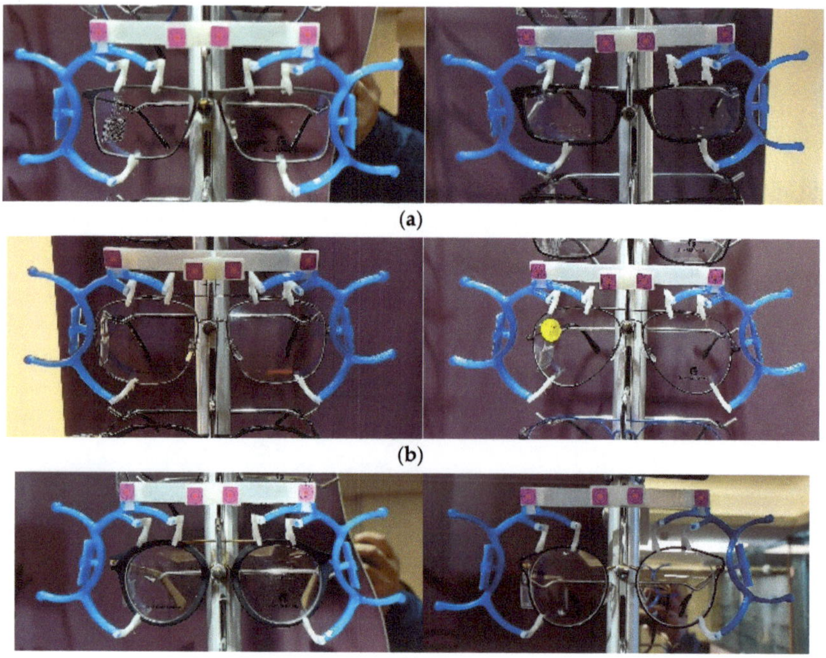

(a)

(b)

(c)

Figure 7. (**a**) "Regular"-shaped glasses frames. (**b**) Large glasses frames in terms of both width and height. (**c**) Round-shaped glasses frames.

Given the good results obtained in testing the marker support system for almost all pairs of glasses tested—with the exception of extremely small or overly large frames, with heights either under 25 mm or above 65 mm—it was concluded that tests could be performed with an actual patient to determine how wearing the supports would influence the measurements taken. While preliminary tests could be performed without a human subject, some parameters could not be simulated—for example, the user might wear the glasses slightly tilted to one side, or certain asymmetries might influence the position of the marker support system in such a way that measurements might be harder to obtain. For this purpose, a human test subject was involved in further investigation, as described in Section 5.

5. Evaluation of the Compliant Mechanism on a Human Patient

In order to confirm that the designed frame would indeed hold its shape when worn by a user and allow for the system to capture certain parameters, tests were performed that involved the device being fixed to a user's glasses, and information was obtained via visual, then computerized, confirmation that the user's parameters were indeed similar to those measured by other means. Such an example is shown in Figure 8a–c, discussed in detail as follows.

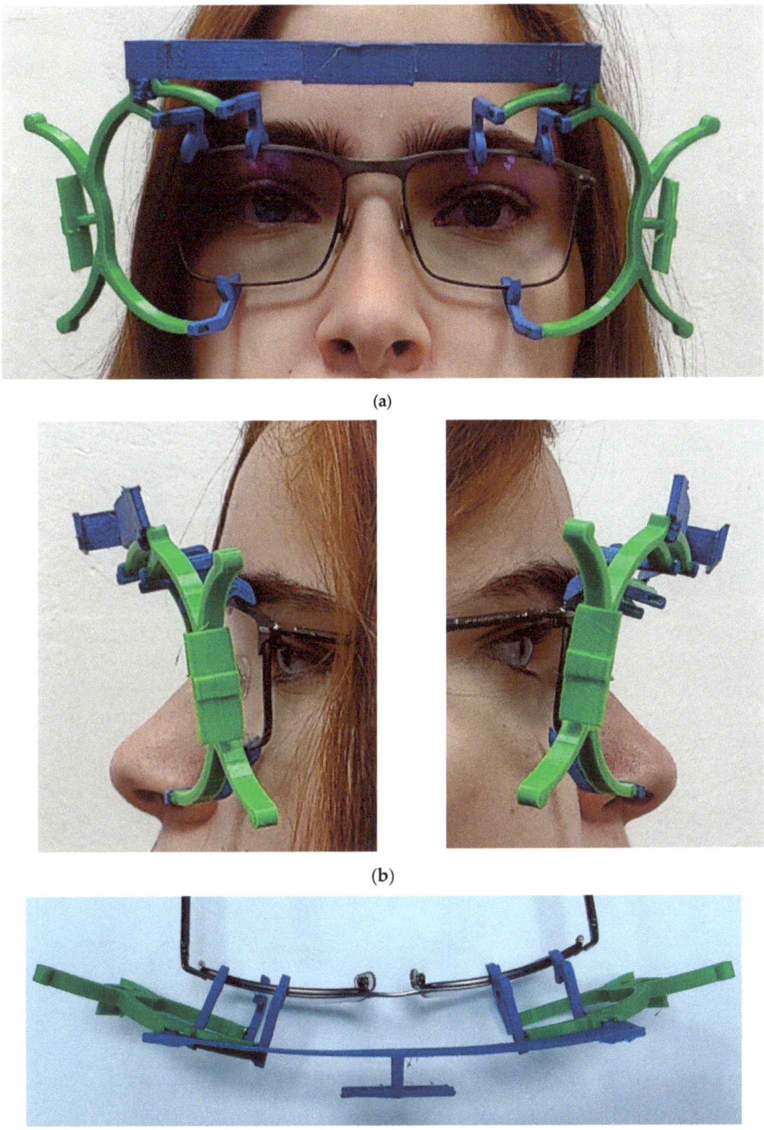

(a)

(b)

(c)

Figure 8. (**a**) Front view of the patient wearing test glasses and the marker support system. (**b**) Lateral view of the patient wearing the glasses and the marker support system. (**c**) Upper view of the glasses with the marker support system.

Figure 8a exhibits a user wearing a "regular" type of glasses frames, along with the marker support system. As can be observed, the supports are not, in any way, inconvenient to the user and allow the optometrist to easily monitor the user's eyes in order to easily monitor for different conditions, such as the squinting that might only occur during specific actions taken by the patient. Since the marker's weight is under 12 g, its effect on the angle of the glasses frames that is relative to the patient is minimal and can be neglected.

Figure 8b allows for a view of the patient wearing the supports along with the glasses frames. This view also allows for confirmation that the markers will, at least visually (to be later confirmed by image processing), allow for an approximation of the user's pantoscopic angle. While it is usual to take only one pantoscopic angle into consideration, the system was designed to allow for different measurements to be taken both for the user's left-side and right-side pantoscopic angle. This view also confirms that, due to the offset of the support system relative to the glasses frames, there is no interaction between the user and the compliant mechanism.

Figure 8c consists of a top-down view of the glasses and compliant mechanism, allowing for confirmation that the curvature of the frames is indeed transferred to the measuring system. Due to the very low force needed to bend the bridge between the two C-shaped main supports, the influence of the marker support system on the curvature of the glasses can be considered non-existent.

As such, it was indeed confirmed that the device mimics the user's pantoscopic angle and the frame's curvature, allowing for an easy measurement of the distance between the lens and the patient's eyes, as well as simpler measurements, such as interpupillary distance, lens size, etc. The methods used to determine these parameters will be described in detail in further work and are the subject of a different side of the research that was undertaken in the creation of the system.

Overall, the mechanism was proven to be easy to use and appropriately sized when mounted on most pairs of glasses frames, with minimal or no effect on the position of the frames relative to the user's face. Also, the support was easy to mount and was in no way inconvenient to the patient.

Using the images captured of the patient wearing the glasses mounted with the marker support system, several tests were conducted to confirm the validity of the assumptions made by the authors during the design process. As such, using a pre-alpha test application, also developed during the work done in this paper (preliminary results have indeed been found to confirm that the measurements taken are close to reality), was conducted by comparing image processing results with those obtained using the usual measurements. Figure 9 depicts the results obtained by analysing an image similar to that in Figure 8a, with markers added in their respective positions.

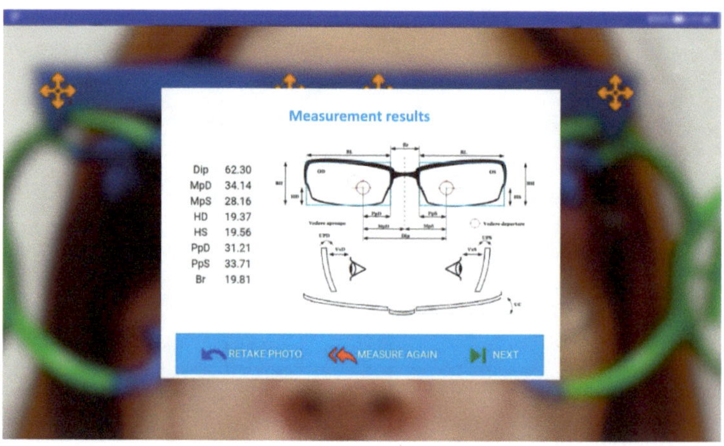

Figure 9. Results obtained during preliminary image recognition measurements.

6. Conclusions

Some of the harder-to-overcome obstacles encountered in the building of these prototypes were shape design, material choice and additive manufacturing techniques to be employed in the manufacturing of the compliant mechanism.

Regarding shape, the design can be split into two separate points to be addressed: one responsible for fixing the support to the frames as well as a bridge that would join the two C-shaped supports. While the initial design of the C-shaped supports was proposed and tested in previous works, adding a bridge introduced a number of issues previously not accounted for: rotation around the Y-axis of the frames, partially compensated by the shape of the joints between the bridge and supports, as well as a larger Y-axis dimension for the bridge, allowing for less rotational movement. The bridge, however, needed to be flexible enough to allow the entire system to follow the curvature of the frames.

The materials used were also scrutinized in terms of weight, ease of use, availability and, last but not least, compatibility with use in close proximity to human skin. While it might be argued that the support itself should not touch the patient at any time, it was considered necessary to guarantee that all the materials used were biologically inert to humans. That being said, while materials such as PLA or TPU, as used in this work, are commonly used around humans, a further scaling or usage of the system with different types of frames might prove to be necessary in order to explore other options.

Following these two choices, a preliminary FEM analysis was performed in order to estimate what could be expected of the mechanism without actually manufacturing it. General estimations performed during this stage were consistent with initial expected results, and this allowed the shape to be tweaked.

The additive technology used for the purposes of this work was FDM, but other candidates might also be considered, such as Digital Light Processing DLP or event Selective Laser Sintering SLS. While the obvious advantage of FDM is its accessibility, high-precision and more advanced materials might require different additive techniques to be used in order to obtain desired results in the mechanical behaviour of a device. There is also the concern of aesthetics—while FDM is precise enough to allow for usability, it is hardly the best in terms of surface quality.

Further work will be performed to design and perfect an application to be used alongside the marker support system in order to obtain measurements. This application will also allow for tests to be made that will further allow for possible modifications to be made to the shape of the part. This application will allow for a mobile computing and image capture device in order to use the markers mounted on the support for determining some parameters relevant to the construction of highly customised progressive lenses. Also, this application will allow for the user's details to be saved in a database and monitored over time, resulting in higher standards in healthcare. This application might even be connected to an online store and might allow users to directly customise their lenses after their measurements have been taken.

While the manufactured and tested marker support system has yielded good results, including in preliminary software tests not depicted in this paper, further extensive measurements need to be made using the system, and a full in-depth evaluation should be performed to assess the viability of the model proposed. There is also a valid point to be made for the pursual, to a specific extent, of a parametric automated design for elastic elements in order for more shapes and sizes of frames to be measured.

The advantages of such a system stem from the fact that small changes can be made to the shapes so that all the models of the frames can be measured using this device. It is also understood that this system takes full advantage of the fact that FDM technologies have advanced and are regularly available in most areas of the world. Long-term, the gathering of measurement data through such a device would allow for certain approximations to be made by means of big data processing and, of course, including the results in the obtention of better and better measurements and more precise prescriptions for patients.

It is expected that this device will allow for more precise, cost-effective measurements to be taken in order to allow for a much better customisation of lenses in general, and progressive lenses in particular, ultimately allowing for better eye healthcare to be brought to a much wider range of patients.

Author Contributions: Conceptualization, V.C.; methodology, V.C., D.B. and B.G.; software, V.C.; validation, E.M., D.B. and D.C.; formal analysis, B.G., D.B. and D.C.; investigation, D.B. and V.C.; resources, B.G., D.B. and E.M.; writing—original draft preparation, V.C., E.M., D.C. and B.G.; writing—review and editing V.C., E.M., D.C. and B.G. All authors have read and agreed to the published version of the manuscript.

Funding: The publication of this paper was funded by the National University of Science and Technology Politehnica Bucharest's PubART project.

Institutional Review Board Statement: Ethical review and approval were waived for this study through POLITEHNICA University of Bucharest Ethics Committee, due to no direct or indirect risk to the test subject as well as no specific rules and regulations for this type of study.

Informed Consent Statement: Informed consent was obtained from all subjects involved in the study. Written informed consent has been obtained from the patients to publish this paper.

Data Availability Statement: Data are contained within the article.

Conflicts of Interest: The authors declare no conflict of interest.

References

1. Constantin, V.; Besnea, D.; Gramescu, B.; Moraru, E. Aspects Related to the Design and Manufacturing of an Original and Innovative Marker Support System for Use in Clinical Optometry. *Appl. Sci.* **2023**, *13*, 2859. [CrossRef]
2. Liaw, C.Y.; Guvendiren, M. Current and emerging applications of 3D printing in medicine. *Biofabrication* **2017**, *9*, 024102 [CrossRef] [PubMed]
3. Dawood, A.; Marti, B.; Sauret-Jackson, V.M.; Darwood, A. 3D printing in dentistry. *Br. Dent. J.* **2015**, *219*, 521–529. [CrossRef]
4. Paul, G.M.; Rezaienia, A.; Wen, P.; Condoor, S.; Parkar, N.; King, W.; Korakianitis, T. Medical applications for 3D printing: Recent developments. *Mo. Med.* **2018**, *115*, 75. [PubMed]
5. Ginestra, P.; Ferraro, R.M.; Zohar-Hauber, K.; Abeni, A.; Giliani, S.; Ceretti, E. Selective laser melting and electron beam melting of Ti6Al4V for orthopedic applications: A comparative study on the applied building direction. *Materials* **2020**, *13*, 5584.
6. Vaish, A.; Vaish, R. 3D printing and its applications in Orthopedics. *J. Clin. Orthop. Trauma* **2018**, *9*, S74–S75. [CrossRef]
7. Ramakrishnan, T.; Schlafly, M.; Reed, K.B. Evaluation of 3D printed anatomically scalable transfemoral prosthetic knee. In Proceedings of the 2017 International Conference on Rehabilitation Robotics (ICORR), London, UK, 17–20 July 2017; IEEE: Piscataway, NJ, USA, 2017; pp. 1160–1164.
8. Garcia, J.; Yang, Z.; Mongrain, R.; Leask, R.L.; Lachapelle, K. 3D printing materials and their use in medical education: A review of current technology and trends for the future. *BMJ Simul. Technol. Enhanc. Learn.* **2018**, *4*, 27. [CrossRef]
9. Tejo-Otero, A.; Buj-Corral, I.; Fenollosa-Artés, F. 3D printing in medicine for preoperative surgical planning: A review. *Ann. Biomed. Eng.* **2020**, *48*, 536–555. [CrossRef]
10. George, M.; Aroom, K.R.; Hawes, H.G.; Gill, B.S.; Love, J. 3D printed surgical instruments: The design and fabrication process. *World J. Surg.* **2017**, *41*, 314–319. [CrossRef]
11. Trenfield, S.J.; Awad, A.; Goyanes, A.; Gaisford, S.; Basit, A.W. 3D printing pharmaceuticals: Drug development to frontline care. *Trends Pharmacol. Sci.* **2018**, *39*, 440–451. [CrossRef]
12. Murphy, S.V.; Atala, A. 3D bioprinting of tissues and organs. *Nat. Biotechnol.* **2014**, *32*, 773–785. [CrossRef] [PubMed]
13. Berglund, G.; Wisniowiecki, A.; Gawedzinski, J.; Applegate, B.; Tkaczyk, T.S. Additive manufacturing for the development of optical/photonic systems and components. *Optica* **2022**, *9*, 623–638. [CrossRef]
14. Ayyildiz, O. Customised spectacles using 3-D printing technology. *Clin. Exp. Optom.* **2018**, *101*, 747–751. [CrossRef] [PubMed]
15. Tsegay, F.; Ghannam, R.; Daniel, N.; Butt, H. 3D Printing Smart Eyeglass Frames: A Review. *ACS Appl. Eng. Mater.* **2023**, *1*, 1142–1163. [CrossRef]
16. Lee, L.; Burnett, A.M.; Panos, J.G.; Paudel, P.; Keys, D.; Ansari, H.M.; Yu, M. 3-D printed spectacles: Potential, challenges and the future. *Clin. Exp. Optom* **2020**, *103*, 590–596. [CrossRef] [PubMed]
17. Solaimani, S.; Parandian, A.; Nabiollahi, N. A holistic view on sustainability in additive and subtractive manufacturing: A comparative empirical study of eyewear production systems. *Sustainability* **2021**, *13*, 10775. [CrossRef]
18. Zhu, Y.; Tang, T.; Zhao, S.; Joralmon, D.; Poit, Z.; Ahire, B.; Keshav, S.; Raje, A.R.; Blair, J.; Zhang, Z.; et al. Recent advancements and applications in 3D printing of functional optics. *Addit. Manuf.* **2022**, *52*, 102682. [CrossRef]
19. Jia, S.; Bu, Y.; Lau, D.S.A.; Lin, Z.; Sun, T.; Lu, W.W.; Lu, S.; Ruan, C.; Chan, C.H.J. Advances in 3D bioprinting technology for functional corneal reconstruction and regeneration. *Front. Bioeng. Biotechnol.* **2022**, *10*, 1065460. [CrossRef]

20. Wang, Y.; Wang, J.; Ji, Z.; Yan, W.; Zhao, H.; Huang, W.; Liu, H. Application of bioprinting in ophthalmology. *Int. J. Bioprinting* **2022**, *8*, 552. [CrossRef]
21. Ruiz-Alonso, S.; Villate-Beitia, I.; Gallego, I.; Lafuente-Merchan, M.; Puras, G.; Saenz-del-Burgo, L.; Pedraz, J.L. Current insights into 3D bioprinting: An advanced approach for eye tissue regeneration. *Pharmaceutics* **2021**, *13*, 308. [CrossRef]
22. Kafle, A.; Luis, E.; Silwal, R.; Pan, H.M.; Shrestha, P.L.; Bastola, A.K. 3D/4D Printing of polymers: Fused deposition modelling (FDM), selective laser sintering (SLS), and stereolithography (SLA). *Polymers* **2021**, *13*, 3101.
23. Szabó, B.; Babuška, I. *Finite Element Analysis: Method, Verification and Validation*, 2nd ed.; Wiley: New York, NY, USA, 2021.
24. David Müzel, S.; Bonhin, E.P.; Guimarães, N.M.; Guidi, E.S. Application of the finite element method in the analysis of composite materials: A review. *Polymers* **2020**, *12*, 818. [CrossRef] [PubMed]
25. Bathe, K.J.; Zhang, H.; Ji, S. Finite element analysis of fluid flows fully coupled with structural interactions. *Comput. Struct.* **1999**, *72*, 1–16. [CrossRef]
26. Liu, X.F.; Wang, Y.; Liu, W.H. Finite element analysis of thermo-mechanical conditions inside the piston of a diesel engine. *Appl. Therm. Eng.* **2017**, *119*, 312–318. [CrossRef]
27. Rajanna, M.R.; Johnson, E.L.; Codoni, D.; Korobenko, A.; Bazilevs, Y.; Liu, N.; Lua, J.; Phan, N.; Hsu, M.C. Finite element methodology for modeling aircraft aerodynamics: Development, simulation, and validation. *Comput. Mech.* **2022**, *70*, 549–563. [CrossRef]
28. Bradai, S.; Naifar, S.; Kanoun, O. Finite element analysis of combined magnetoelectric-electrodynamic vibration energy converter. *J. Phys. Conf. Ser.* **2015**, *660*, 012111. [CrossRef]
29. Wang, T.; Green, R.; Guldiken, R.; Wang, J.; Mohapatra, S.; Mohapatra, S.S. Finite element analysis for surface acoustic wave device characteristic properties and sensitivity. *Sensors* **2019**, *19*, 1749. [CrossRef]
30. Abueidda, D.W.; Elhebeary, M.; Shiang, C.S.A.; Pang, S.; Al-Rub, R.K.A.; Jasiuk, I.M. Mechanical properties of 3D printed polymeric Gyroid cellular structures: Experimental and finite element study. *Mater. Des.* **2019**, *165*, 107597. [CrossRef]
31. Castaldo, P.; Gino, D.; Mancini, G. Safety formats for non-linear finite element analysis of reinforced concrete structures: Discussion, comparison and proposals. *Eng. Struct.* **2019**, *193*, 136–153. [CrossRef]
32. Nurhaniza, M.; Ariffin, M.K.A.; Ali, A.; Mustapha, F.; Noraini, A.W. Finite element analysis of composites materials for aerospace applications. *IOP Conf. Ser. Mater. Sci. Eng.* **2010**, *11*, 012010. [CrossRef]
33. Purohit, R.; Khitoliya, P.; Koli, D.K. Design and finite element analysis of an automotive clutch assembly. *Procedia Mater. Sci.* **2014**, *6*, 490–502. [CrossRef]
34. Soro, N.; Brassart, L.; Chen, Y.; Veidt, M.; Attar, H.; Dargusch, M.S. Finite element analysis of porous commercially pure titanium for biomedical implant application. *Mater. Sci. Eng. A* **2018**, *725*, 43–50. [CrossRef]
35. Cicciù, M. Bioengineering methods of analysis and medical devices: A current trends and state of the art. *Materials* **2020**, *13*, 797. [CrossRef] [PubMed]
36. Ramasubramanian, V.S.; Meenatchi Sundaram, S.; Thomas, R.; Ramesh, S.V.; Raghuvir Pai, B.; Hazarika, M.; Abdul Khader, S.M.; Poojary, R.G.; Girish, H.; Crasto, V.S. Finite element analysis of cornea and lid wiper during blink, with and without contact lens. *J. Ophthalmol.* **2022**, *2022*, 7930334. [CrossRef] [PubMed]
37. Moraru, E. Research on the Realization of Dental Prostheses by Selective Laser Deposition and Other Additive Technologies. Ph.D. Thesis, Politehnica University of Bucharest, Bucharest, Romania, 2021. (In Romanian).
38. Besnea, D.; Rizescu, C.I.; Rizescu, D.; Comeaga, D.; Ciobanu, R.; Moraru, E. Study of deflection behaviour of 3D printed leaf springs. In Proceedings of the 8th International Conference on Advanced Concepts in Mechanical Engineering, Iasi, Romania, 7–8 June 2018; Volume 444, p. 042008.
39. Mohamed, O.A.; Masood, S.H.; Bhowmik, J.L. Optimization of fused deposition modeling process parameters: A review of current research and future prospects. *Adv. Manuf.* **2015**, *3*, 42–53.
40. Solomon, I.J.; Sevvel, P.; Gunasekaran, J. A review on the various processing parameters in FDM. *Mater. Today Proc.* **2021**, *37*, 509–514.
41. Dey, A.; Yodo, N. A systematic survey of FDM process parameter optimization and their influence on part characteristics. *J. Manuf. Mater. Process.* **2019**, *3*, 64.
42. Enemuoh, E.U.; Duginski, S.; Feyen, C.; Menta, V.G. Effect of process parameters on energy consumption, physical, and mechanical properties of fused deposition modeling. *Polymers* **2021**, *13*, 2406

applied sciences

MDPI

Article

Mechatronic Device Used to Evaluate the Performance of a Compliant Mechanism and Image Processing System in Determining Optometric Parameters

Victor Constantin, Daniel Comeagă, Bogdan Grămescu, Daniel Besnea, Adrian Cartal * and Edgar Moraru

Department of Mechatronics and Precision Mechanics, Faculty of Mechanical Engineering and Mechatronics, National University of Science and Technology POLITEHNICA Bucharest, 060042 Bucharest, Romania; edgar.moraru@upb.ro (E.M.)

* Correspondence: adrian.cartal@upb.ro

Abstract: The work presented in the paper describes a mechatronic test stand and technique employed to determine the accuracy of a system developed by the authors to assist optometrists in measuring parameters used in the customization of progressive lenses, as well as regular lenses. The system aims to offer information about interpupillary distance, pantoscopic angle, and vertex distance, as well as measurements useful in correctly mounting the lenses in the frames. This is conducted by attaching a marker support system to the user's frame and determining the user's dimensions by using image acquisition techniques performed via a custom application built for this purpose. In this paper, a test mannequin is used to determine the accuracy of the system, with measurements being compared to those obtained by using classic methods. This method is used to determine the accuracy of the measurements in a controlled environment. Following the good results obtained in this paper and pending some improvements to the application, clinical tests will be performed on a small scale in selected optometrist offices.

Keywords: mechatronic system; characterization; optometry; automatic testing

1. Introduction

The present work represents a logical continuation of the research developed by the authors in the previously published papers [1,2] that refer to the complaint system executed by additive technologies with possible uses in the field of personalized clinical optometry. The first paper [1] is mainly based on the design and technology of obtaining an important part of the proposed system-compliant mechanism for marker support, which directly fastens the glasses. Following the research carried out, several constructive options were proposed for the mechanism, and in the end, the optimal geometry was chosen for the given application, taking into account the anatomical, technical, and other important aspects that can intervene and complicate the process of use and/or may possibly affect the correctness of the data obtained during use. The choice of the optimal materials and technology for obtaining the structures was also discussed, and justified-thermoplastic materials and respectively Fused Deposition Modeling (FDM) technology from the family of additive manufacturing were chosen. The choice of technology is mainly due to the following considerations: the ease of use of the technology, the possibility of obtaining complicated and personalized geometries in a relatively short time, and, at the same time, the low production cost. Regarding the materials for the compliant mechanism, usual thermoplastic materials used in FDM technology were proposed (PLA (Polylactic acid), ABS (Acrylonitrile Butadiene Styrene), and TPU (Thermoplastic polyurethane)) based on their adequate mechanical properties and availability. The sizing of the compliant mechanism was based on the standards used in optometry regarding the dimensions of spectacle frames and the lenses before they were cut and adjusted in the frames. In order to evaluate the displacement by applying the necessary force and implicitly the opening of the gripping elements for fastening the glasses, a study was also carried out using the finite element method, after which the mechanical behavior of the compliant mechanism was estimated, and mechanical characteristics were determined such as the degree of displacement, von Mises stress and equivalent strain for the three thermoplastic materials proposed, comparing their mechanical performances of the materials when applying certain loads. Furthermore, a comparative discussion about the 3D printed parts obtained by FDM technology from three thermoplastic materials used and their 3D printing conditions and parameters was addressed in the paper [1]; the authors also proposed an electro-pneumatic experimental rig for testing 3D printed compliant mechanisms for marker supports.

The second paper of the authors [2] approaches the continuation, development, and deepening of the studies in the first article and refers to the design and testing of the fully compliant mechanism for complex personalized lenses in the field of clinical optometry. In this study, the component elements that govern the interesting mechanical behavior of the structures are introduced, as well as the optometric parameters that can be measured and determined with the help of the developed compliant mechanisms: interpupillary distance (both left and right), lens width (both left and right), lens height, bridge width, pupil distance to lower part of the lens and so on. Also, mechanical analysis using finite element method tools was performed for the fully compliant system in order to estimate the behavior of the structure in the function of applied loads of work conditions for a certain type of glasses before the execution of the mechanisms and to determine mechanical characteristics of interest. Finally, the second study discusses the manufacturing testing of developed different types of glasses, preliminarily evaluates the compliant mechanism on a human patient, and presents the results obtained during the first image recognition determination.

Figure 1 [1,2] shows the graphical summary and synthesis regarding the research subjects of previous papers of the authors. The first case (left part of the figure) is about the design, simulation, manufacturing, and testing of one of the most important components of the mechanical structure of the system-grasping element [1], and the second paper discussed similar things about the complete system of compliant mechanism (right part of the figure) [2]. As shown in Figure 2, the complete system of the proposed compliant mechanism consists mainly of several sections that allow the positioning of the marker support (MS) sections in view of the measurements of interest of the specific optometric parameters and the grasping mechanisms that practically fix the glasses to be investigated. More details about the working principle and the mechanical behavior of the complete compliant mechanism can be found in the previous paper of the authors [2].

The system supports the placement of markers in relation to a user's face, enabling the determination of specific dimensions based on the user's facial features and selected glasses frames. These dimensions include pupillary and interpupillary distance, glasses frame curvature, pantoscopic angle on each side of the user's face, and measurements required for customizing the lens to fit the frames [3]. The markers, made of specific-colored adhesive low-gloss paper, are positioned with a custom stencil to ensure accuracy. A chart in Figure 3 illustrates the measurements possible with this system. By capturing close-up and distant photos of the patient wearing the glasses and marker support setup, all necessary parameters can be accurately determined.

Some of the measurements that can be obtained include the following:

- Interpupillary Distance (IDR) which consists of total, right, and left measurements
- Lens Width (LW) for both the left and right lenses
- Lens Height (LH) for the left and right lenses
- Bridge Width (BW)
- Distance from the pupils to the lower part of the lens (BHR and BHL)
- Pupil distance to the lower part of the lens for both eyes (BIL and BIR)
- Vertex Distance (VL and VD)
- Distance between the pupil and the lens (PAR and PAL)

- Pantoscopic Angle Right (PAR) and Pantoscopic Angle Left (PAL)
- Glasses frame curvature (FC)

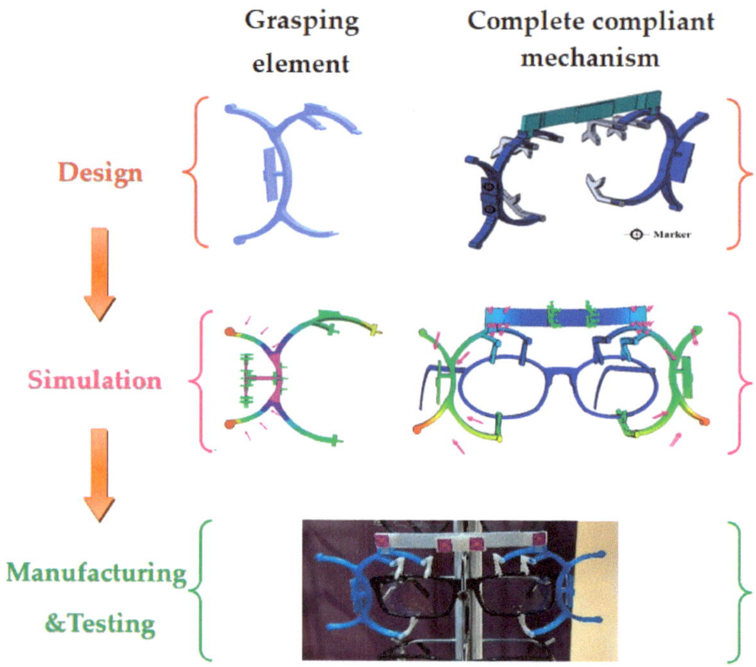

Figure 1. Graphical summary of previous research of the authors regarding the approached subject [1,2].

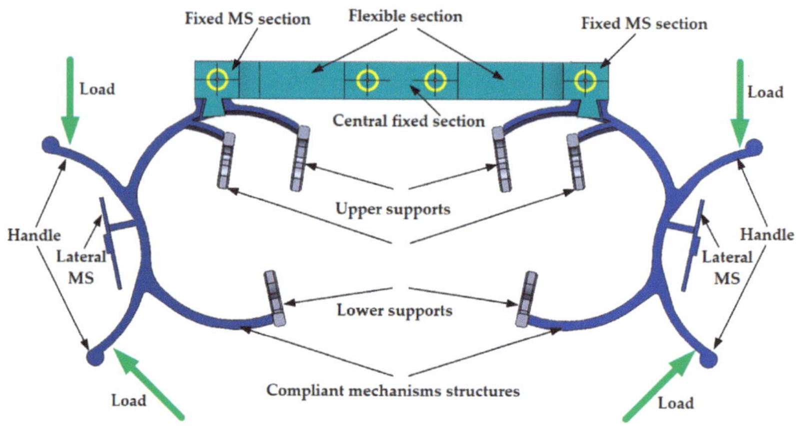

Figure 2. Geometry and key elements of developed complete compliant mechanism for optometric field [2].

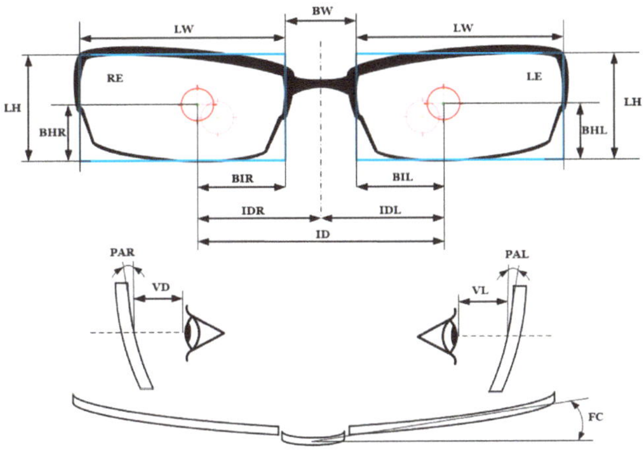

Figure 3. Measurements taken by the system [2].

Recent advancements in the optical and optometric fields, driven by additive technologies [4], have enabled the creation of personalized glass frames through additive manufacturing [5–7]. This development marks the beginning of a transformative era in optometry, allowing for highly customized frames. Selective laser deposition technology, using metal or polymeric powders, has proven efficient in producing these frames with minimal waste. Additionally, additive technologies facilitate the production of various lenses and multifunctional components, enhancing optical systems and devices [8,9]. In ophthalmology, bioprinting techniques for corneal reconstruction and other eye tissues are showing promising results in advanced testing phases, offering significant future benefits [10,11].

3D printing in medicine enables the creation of customized implants, prosthetics, and surgical tools tailored to individual patients. It facilitates bioprinting for tissue and organ regeneration, such as corneal and cartilage reconstruction. This technology enhances precision in medical procedures, accelerates innovation, and significantly improves patient outcomes. This can be easily paired with image acquisition techniques that involve capturing detailed images of the eye using technologies like OCT (Optical Coherence Tomography), fundus photography, and corneal topography [12–15]. These images help diagnose and monitor eye conditions, assess retinal health, and guide treatments, ensuring accurate and effective patient care. This can be easily paired with the field of mechatronics, which integrates robotics, electronics, and computer control for advanced surgical tools, diagnostic devices, and patient care automation.

Considering the lines discussed above, the present paper aims to continue the research topic by the authors, namely to conceive and develop a mechatronic rig device for the testing and measuring the specific optometric parameters with the help of the complete compliant mechanism in order to collect and to process the data obtained in the function of some technical aspects of the measurements and to correct and choose the optimal measurement conditions for possible implementation and use of this solution in clinical and practical optometry.

In this paper, a semi-automatic test bench was built to allow the authors to test out the marker support system and application proposed previously on a mannequin, starting from known dimensions. This allows for a comparison to be made between classic methods of obtaining key parameters as opposed to those obtained by means of the application proposed in this paper. In this stage, the setup allows for testing of the method without having to take into account the patient's movement. Also, the system allows for a very large number of measurements to be taken of the same subject–impossible with a human patient.

2. Mechatronic Testing Device Design and Construction

In order to allow the apparatus to be tested, as well as calibrated for real-life measurements, a test bench was designed and manufactured. The basic schematic for this is shown in Figures 4 and 5. A mannequin head (3) is placed on a rotary platform (4) connected to a stepper motor. This allows for movement in three increments: at 0, 90, and 180 degrees, with the 90-degree position corresponding to the patient facing the tablet's camera (1) while the other two positions correspond to the user looking left and right. The assembly is placed on a screw-driven linear axis (5 and 6), actuated by using a second stepper motor (8). This allows the head to be placed at various distance increments relative to the camera of the tablet and allows the impact of said distance on the measurements to be viewed. The distances chosen are between 50 and 100 cm, with a 10 cm increment. These were chosen to allow for the subject to be in full view of the camera at the closest range and the maximum distance at which the markers (2) are still detected by the application. The tablet is placed on a fixed support (9) that allows for the best in-focus position (10) of the camera relative to the mannequin's head. The entire assembly is placed on a support plate (7).

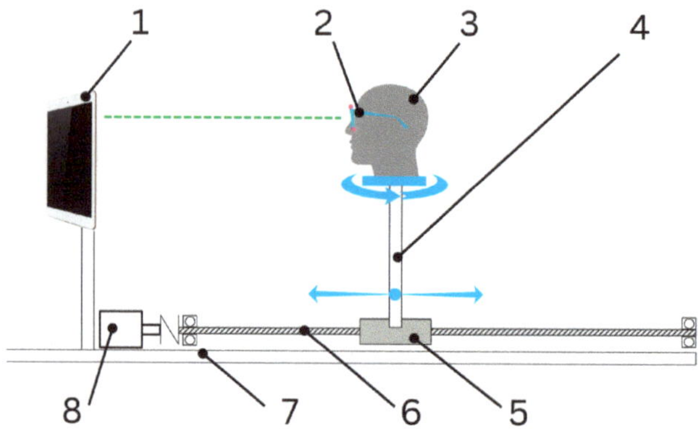

Figure 4. Basic schematic of the test stand, side view.

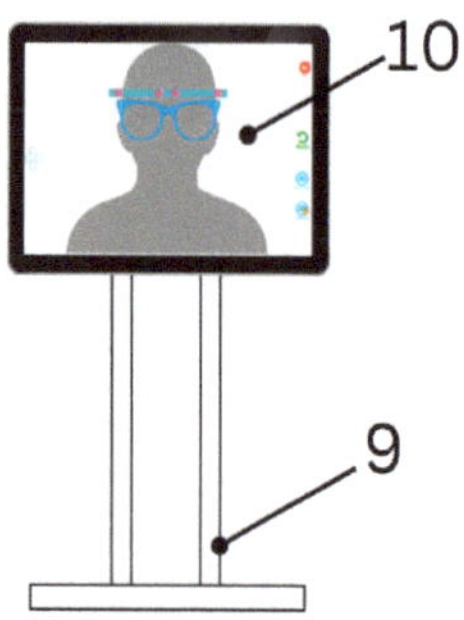

Figure 5. Basic schematic of the test stand, front.

The proposed system was designed using 3D software and assembled using a standard 20 mm × 20 mm aluminum extruded profile, along with connectors and t-slot fastening elements (Figure 6). Stepper motors used are common Nema 23 standard, along with TB6560 drivers and ESP32 microcontrollers. Head positioning is conducted in an open loop, while the linear axis is equipped with end stops.

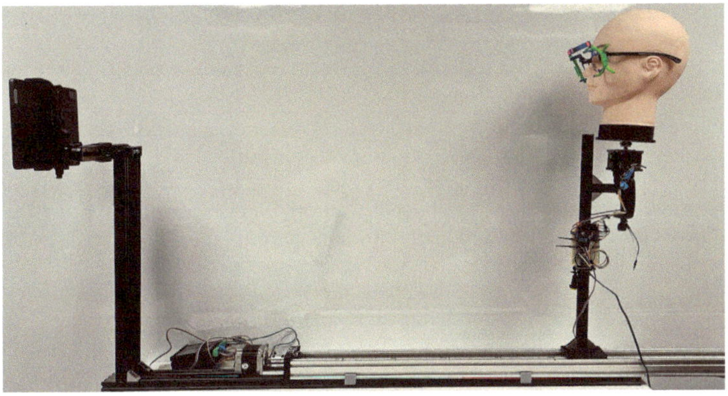

Figure 6. Mechatronic test bench, side view.

The designed system allows faster measurements to be taken since a human is no longer involved, through automation of certain steps, but also for much better repeatability and an overall lower level of errors. This also allowed us to determine what part of the errors was due to human interaction with the system.

A total of three images can be captured using the device (Figure 7): one front and one for each side of the test mannequin. The measurements that can be taken from this are explained in Table 1.

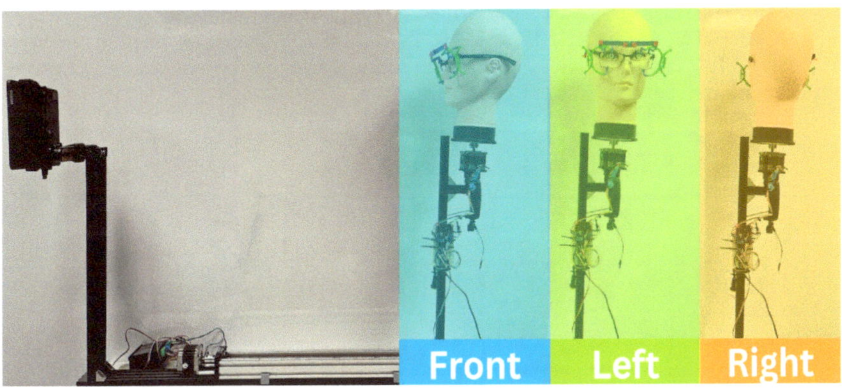

Figure 7. Overview of the test stand.

Table 1. Optometric parameters that can be taken by measurements.

Image Step/Stepper Motor Angle	Parameters
Front/0 degrees	Interpupillary Distance, Semi-pupillary distance left and right, Frame curvature, Lens height and width
Left/+90 degrees	Pantoscopic angle left, Vertex distance left
Right/−90 degrees	Pantoscopic angle right, Vertex distance right

3. Methodology Used for Measurements

The application to be used is developed solely for this purpose and features elements that will allow the optometrist to explain the functionality of specific lens types, measure the patient's parameters using the software and marker frame, order lenses, and other activities specific to their work, beyond the scope of this paper. As such, the paper will focus only on the measurement aspects and will only briefly mention the other parts of the application.

The measurement module of the application allows for two modes of acquisition using two different measurement modules. These are:

- Simple measurements: allowing for interpupillary distance and semi-pupillary distance for each eye. Along with these, measurements for the bridge of the frames, lens mounting height, lateral parameters (pupillary height), and lens width and height will be performed in this stage. This is performed for both far and close mounting of the glasses so as to allow for customization of the final, regarding the different parameters typically obtained in each case.
- Complex measurements: These complete measurements also allow for vertex distance acquisition (distance from the pupil to the lens's plane) as well as pantoscopic angle for each side of the patient (left and right). Two measurements are taken to allow for maximum customization of both the frames and progressive lenses.

The steps taken in each of the two measuring modes are presented in Figures 8 and 9.

With the system in the reference position (distance of 50 cm from the tablet, mannequin in front position), a frontal image is captured, and automatic marker recognition is performed (Figure 10), followed by a boxing stage in which the edges of the glasses frames are identified. This allows for measurements corresponding to Image Step 1 from Table 1 to be acquired. Following this stage, the head is rotated 90 degrees to the left for Step 2 (Figure 11). Following automatic marker recognition and measurements (pantoscopic angle and vertex), the head is again rotated in the opposite direction, 180 degrees. Acquisition of images relevant to Step 3 is performed, and measurements are taken. Even though automatic color marker recognition and pupil recognition are automatic, some adjustments are necessary and are performed by a human operator. The steps are repeated for a number of 50 measurements, and then the mannequin is moved 10 cm further away from the tablet. The previous steps are then redone, and the results are logged into the application's database.

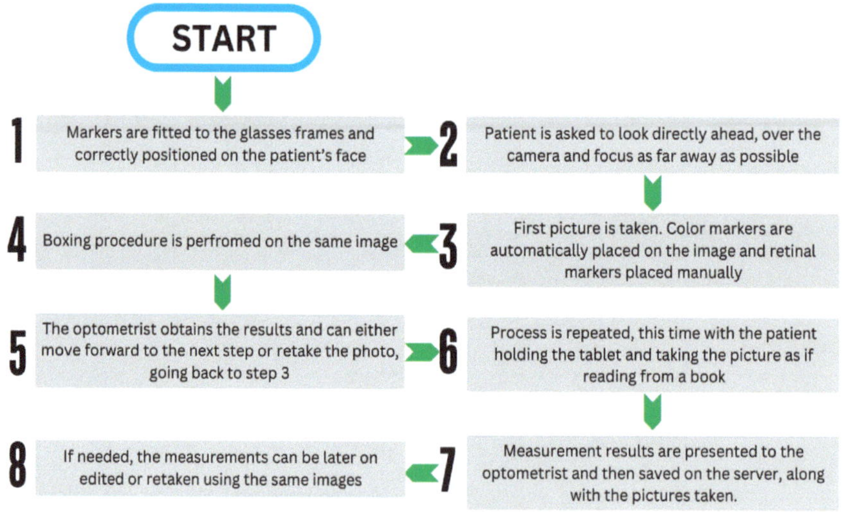

Figure 8. Simple measurements logic diagram.

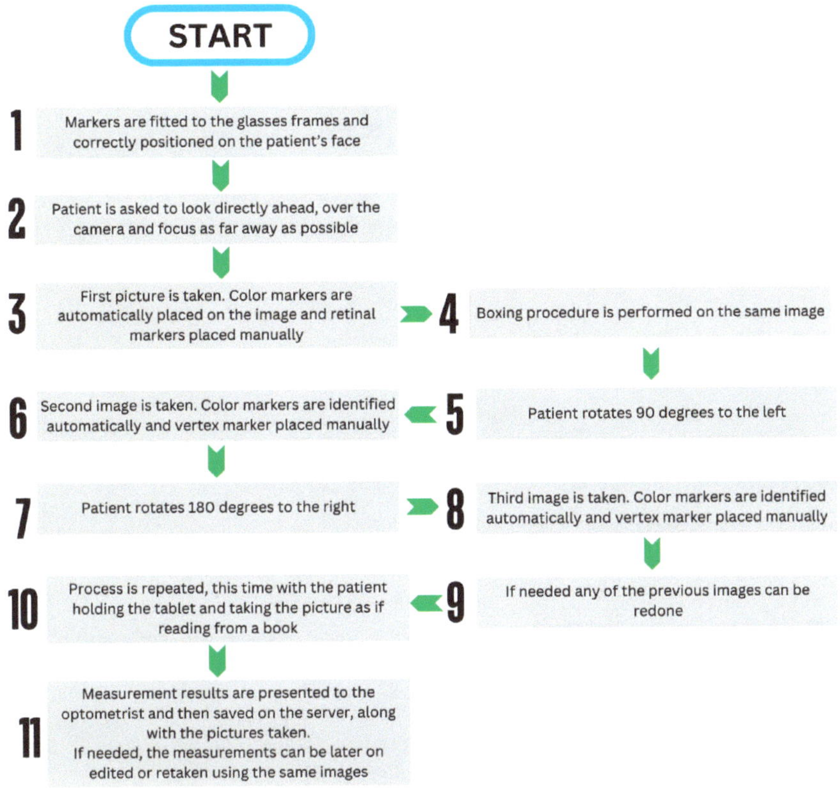

Figure 9. Complex measurements logic diagram.

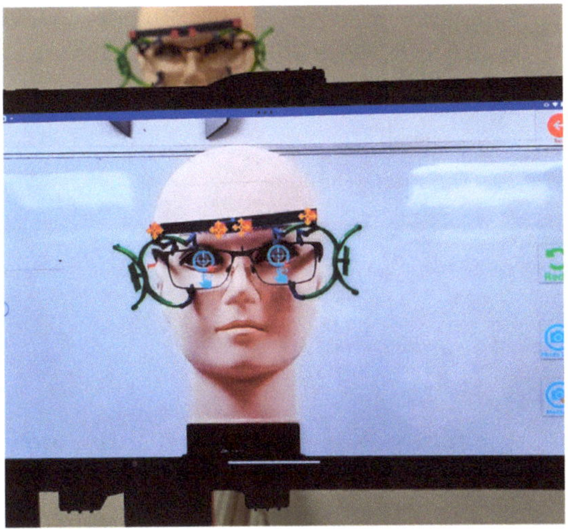

Figure 10. Frontal measurements automatic color and eye recognition.

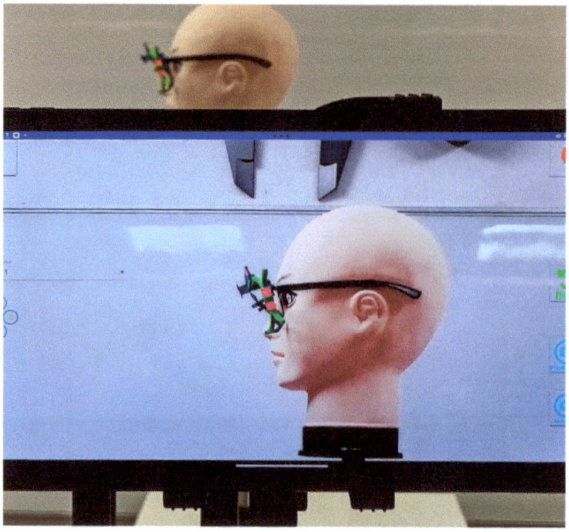

Figure 11. Side image automatic marker recognition.

4. Results and Discussion

The proposed system was tested in the following conditions:

- Measurements were taken by an optometrist with no previous experience with the application. Also, the optometrist was not given any information about the algorithm used to determine the measured parameters so as not to influence the final result. In addition to this, the real measurements were not communicated to the operator prior to finishing the measurement cycle. Initial data is obtained by measuring the distances and angles using basic methods: rulers and protactors.
- A total of approximately 50 measurements was taken for each point along the x-axis, at 50, 60, 70, 80, 90, and 100 cm. Each measurement consisted of one frontal, one right, and one left image. An average total of 150 images was captured and interpreted at 50 cm before moving on to 60 cm and so on.
- In total, over 300 measurements were taken, with over 900 images interpreted in total.
- Actual mannequin measurements are as follows:
  - Interpupillary distance (ID): 51.5 mm
  - Semi-distance left (IDL): 26.5 mm
  - Semi-distance right (IDR): 25 mm
  - Pantoscopic angle (PA): 8 degrees
  - Vertex distance (VD): 11.5 mm

In the following part of the paper, the results obtained after the measurements are presented and discussed as needed.

As previously mentioned, the results were determined for the interpupillary distance (total (ID) and semi-distances (IDL and IDR)), pantoscopic angle, and vertex distance depending on the distance to the target and compared with the real data.

The data obtained was interpreted in graphic form both for individual distances to the target and concatenated in order to compare the dispersion of the results on all the distances to the target approached. In addition, average measured distance, average absolute error (modulus of the difference between the measured data and the real data), and standard deviations for all parameters of interest were calculated and presented in graphic and tabular form.

During the measurements, each set of data was uploaded individually to an online private database and later downloaded for processing. The data revealed a clear difference between taking the measurements at different distances from the mannequin, with absolute errors increasing for interpupillary distance from an average of 0.5 mm to over 2 mm, as shown in Figures 12 and 13.

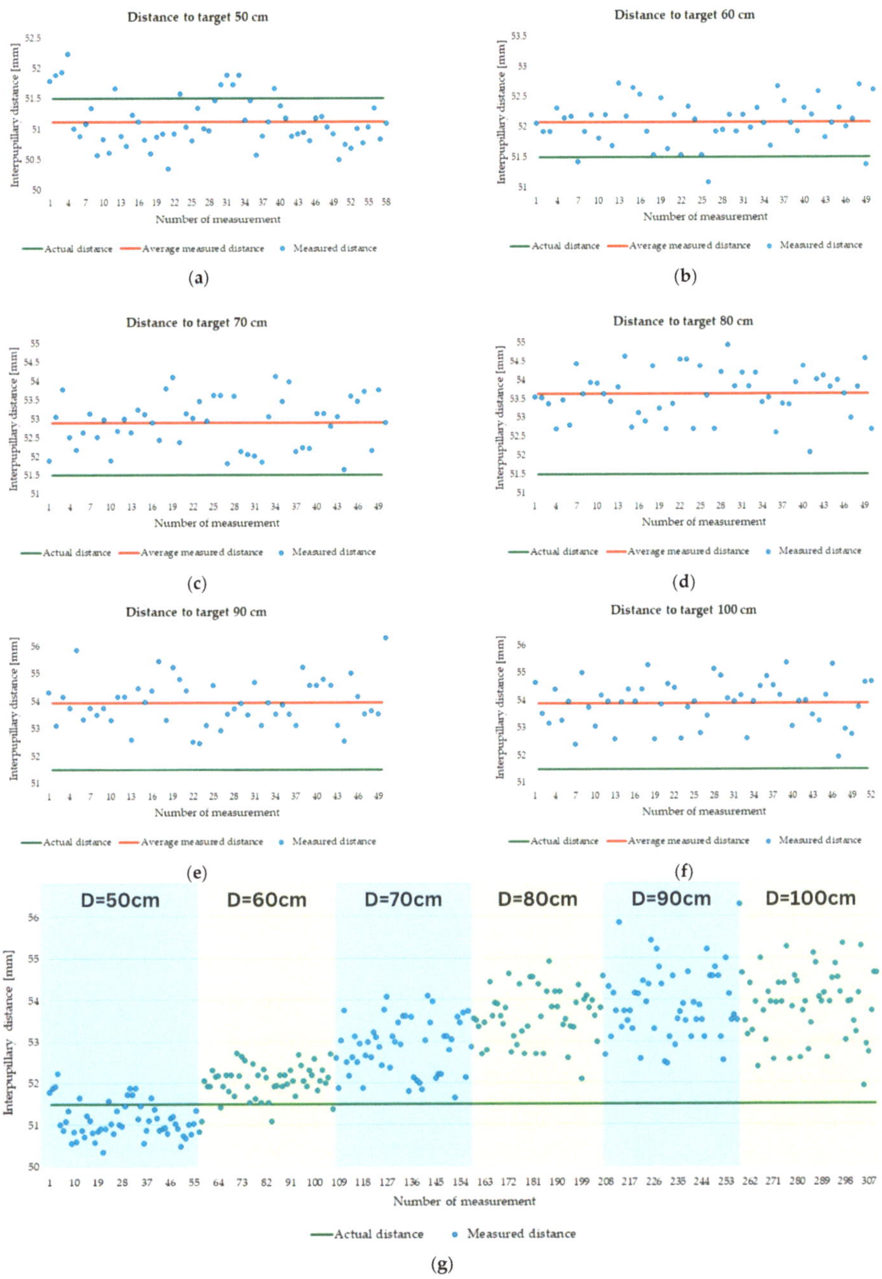

Figure 12. (**a**) Interpupillary measurement at 50 cm; (**b**) Interpupillary measurement at 60 cm; (**c**) Interpupillary measurement at 70 cm; (**d**) Interpupillary measurement at 80 cm; (**e**) Interpupillary measurement at 90 cm; (**f**) Interpupillary measurement at 100 cm; (**g**) Comparison chart of error distribution obtained for interpupillary distance.

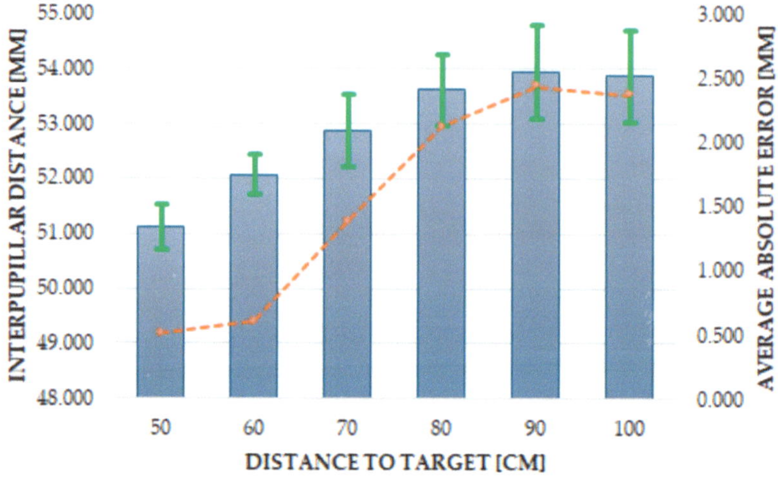

Figure 13. Comparative analysis of obtained results regarding the interpupillary distance measurement.

A detailed description of the errors at each distance was needed, as shown in Figure 12a–f. Each of these graphs shows the actual average distance measured as line plots, as well as the actual measured distance as points in each of the charts.

To further allow a trend to be observed, a general chart of the measurements was plotted, as shown in Figure 12g. There is a clear increase in error over 70 cm, with the error increasing the further the mannequin is from the tablet.

In the current case, the absolute errors for each distance could be attributed to the movement of the camera by the optometrist during image acquisition or errors in image recognition (color and pupillary markers).

Interpupillary distance measurement has also produced the semi-pupillary distance, the distance between the center of the mannequin's face and pupil. These measurements were also plotted in graphs shown in Figure 14a–f, with a concatenated view in the graph shown in Figure 14g. The same behavior can be observed as the absolute error increases with lower precision in the obtained images.

The pantoscopic angle is the tilt of eyeglass lenses towards the cheeks, enhancing vision and comfort. Vertex distance is the space between the back of the lens and the front of the eye. Both are crucial for optimal lens performance, affecting visual clarity and prescription accuracy.

As stated previously, measurements were also performed for the pantoscopic angle as well as the vertex distance (distance between the pupil and the plane of the lens). Results have shown that similar to interpupillary measurements, vertex distance is affected by the distance at which the images are captured. This is shown in the other measurements discussed further in the paper. The behavior is best observed in the latter, with the measurements "drifting" towards lower values, with the increase in distance between the tablet and the markers.

However, very little, if any, effect of distance over the pantoscopic angle was observed. Regarding these measurements, since the mannequin does not feature any asymmetrical characteristics, the measurements were considered identical for each side. These are also shown in Figure 16a–f for each distance, along with Figure 16g, which offers a general overview of the trend in the obtained values.

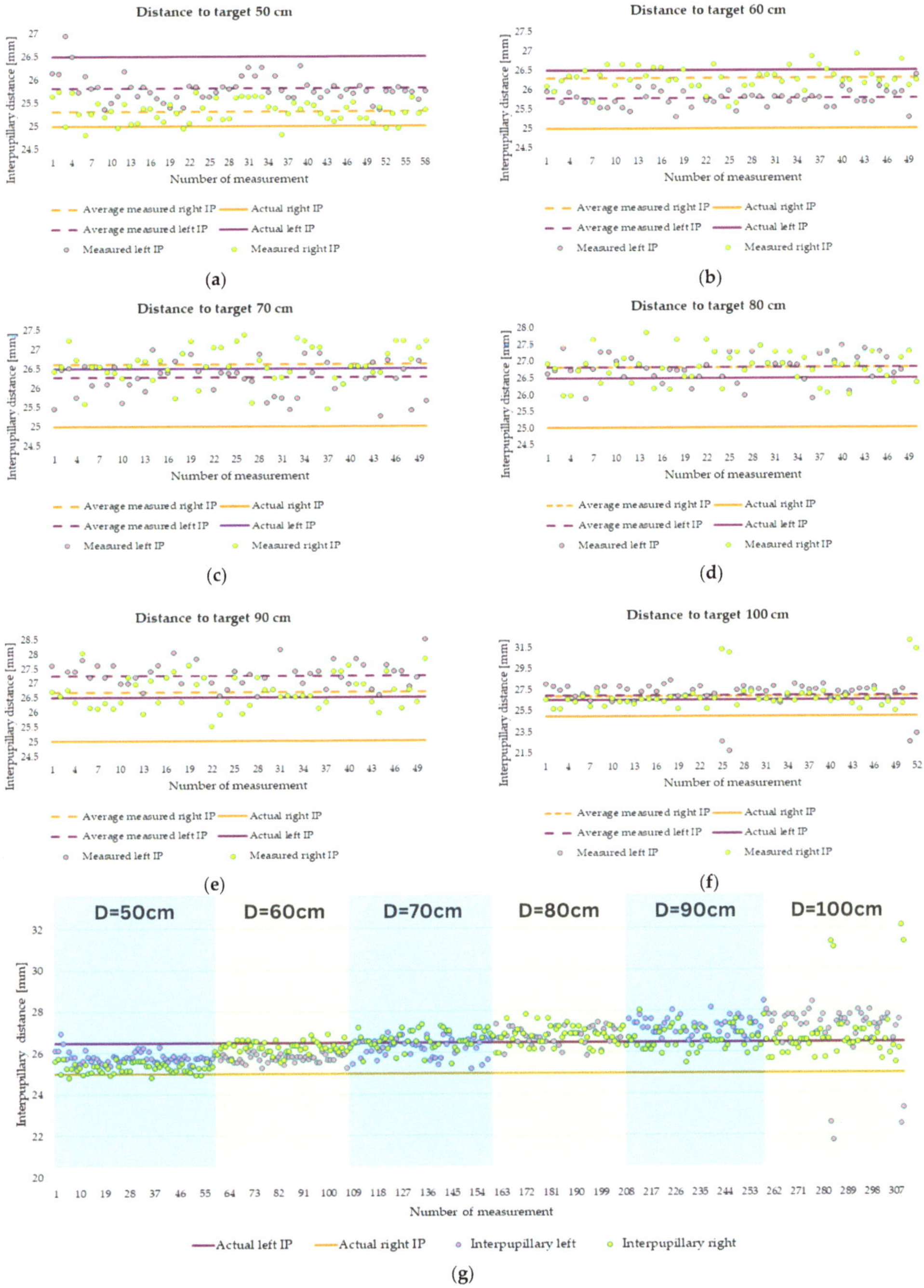

Figure 14. (**a**) Interpupillary measurement at 50 cm; (**b**) Interpupillary measurement at 60 cm; (**c**) Interpupillary measurement at 70 cm; (**d**) Interpupillary measurement at 80 cm; (**e**) Interpupillary measurement at 90 cm; (**f**) Interpupillary measurement at 100 cm; (**g**) Comparison chart of error distribution obtained for interpupillary distance.

The following will present the main interpretations and findings resulting from the experimental determinations according to the obtained parameters.

Analyzing the graphs in Figures 12 and 13 and Table 2, it is clearly seen how the measured average ID increases and deviates from reality as the distance to the target increases. The same general tendency can be observed in the case of average absolute errors and standard deviations. Therefore, for a distance of 50 cm from the target, the following data were obtained for the interpupillary distance: average measured distance of 51.115 mm with a standard deviation (SD) of 0.416 and with maximum and minimum values of 52.23 mm and of 50.34 mm, respectively and absolute average error from the actual distance of 0.503 mm, appearing to be the most optimal distance from the target among those investigated for the correctness of the measurements of this parameter. If at 60 cm to target, the deviations from reality do not seem to increase significantly, being comparable to those at 50 cm, starting with a distance to target of 70 cm, the results of the measurements become more and more distant from the actual data, for example at 90 and 100 cm to target, having an average absolute error of 2.438 mm and 2.374 mm, almost five times higher compared to a distance of 50 cm to target. Regarding the determined semi-distances ((IDL and IDR) Figures 14 and 15 and Tables 3 and 4), it was found, in general, a greater predisposition to errors for IDR—starting with a distance of 60 cm to target—the average absolute errors exceed 1.25 mm (for IDL, the average absolute error exceeds 1 mm compared to the real data only for the distance of 100 cm to target). Also, at a distance of 100 cm, some significantly different results appear compared to the rest of the measurements, this being visible on the graphs in Figure 14f,g through the points further away from the rest of the data–very large distance to target representing an amplification of possible errors caused by the human factor.

Table 2. Obtained data for interpupillary distance measurement.

Distance to Target [cm]	Actual Distance [mm]	Average Measured Distance ± SD [mm]	Average Absolute Error [mm]	Maximum Value [mm]	Minimum Value [mm]
50	51.5	51.115 ± 0.416	0.503	52.23	50.34
60		52.073 ± 0.366	0.598	52.73	51.09
70		52.881 ± 0.669	1.381	54.11	51.65
80		53.621 ± 0.643	2.121	54.92	52.09
90		53.938 ± 0.851	2.438	56.29	52.46
100		53.874 ± 0.826	2.374	55.35	51.92

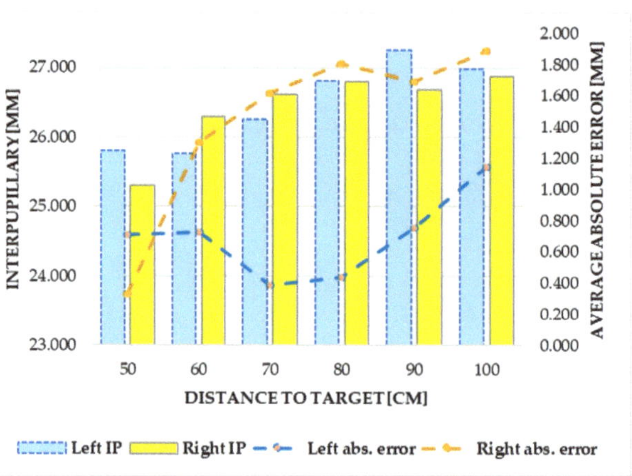

Figure 15. Comparative analysis of obtained results regarding the interpupillary distance measurements (left and right).

Table 3. Obtained data for interpupillary distance measurement (left).

Distance to Target [cm]	Actual Distance [mm]	Average Measured Distance ± SD [mm]	Average Absolute Error [mm]	Maximum Value [mm]	Minimum Value [mm]
50	26.5	25.806 ± 0.286	0.710	26.94	25.34
60		25.774 ± 0.220	0.726	26.38	25.27
70		26.266 ± 0.451	0.384	27.00	25.25
80		26.815 ± 0.415	0.438	27.46	25.88
90		27.252 ± 0.447	0.752	28.48	26.53
100		26.989 ± 1.406	1.142	28.42	21.73

Table 4. Obtained data for interpupillary distance measurement (right).

Distance to Target [cm]	Actual Distance [mm]	Average Measured Distance ± SD [mm]	Average Absolute Error [mm]	Maximum Value [mm]	Minimum Value [mm]
50	25	25.309 ± 0.239	0.330	25.75	24.81
60		26.298 ± 0.291	1.298	26.92	25.56
70		26.616 ± 0.465	1.616	27.38	25.46
80		26.806 ± 0.471	1.806	27.85	25.98
90		26.688 ± 0.555	1.688	28.04	25.52
100		26.885 ± 1.423	1.885	32.11	25.50

When it comes to the pantoscopic angle (Figures 16 and 17 and Table 5), there is generally a tendency to decrease the measured angle and move away from the real angle when the distance to the target increases. The closest results to reality this time, too, are obtained for the distance to the target of 50 cm. The distance to the target for measuring the pantoscopic angle does not greatly affect the dispersion of the results compared to the obtained averages nor the average absolute errors up to a distance to the target of 80 cm (inclusive); the visible differences in the absolute errors becoming apparent at 90 cm and 100 cm to target. Finally, vertex distance measurements (Figures 18 and 19 and Table 6) confirm that the distance of 50 cm to the target is the most suitable for performing the measurements in terms of accordance with the actual data. With the increase of the distance to the target, a successive increase of the vertex distance and a distance from the actual vertex up to a distance to the target of 90 cm can be observed, at the same time increasing the average absolute errors. However, the deviations from the average obtained for the measured values are located in an approximately comparable range for all the distances involved in the experimental research to determine the vertex distance.

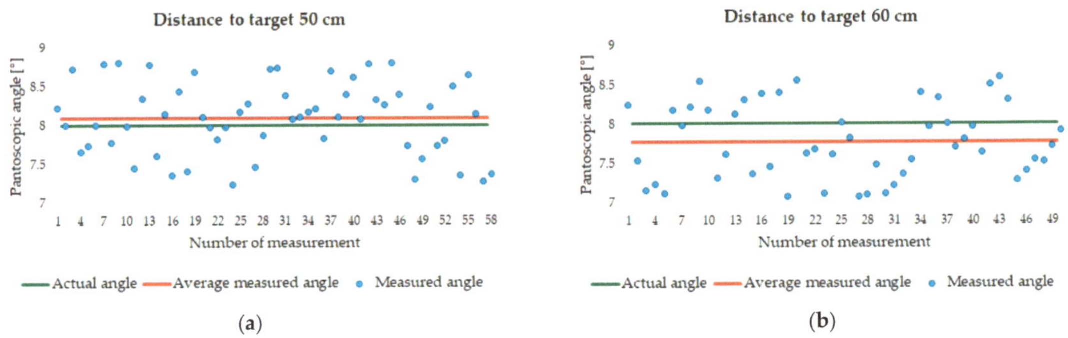

Figure 16. *Cont.*

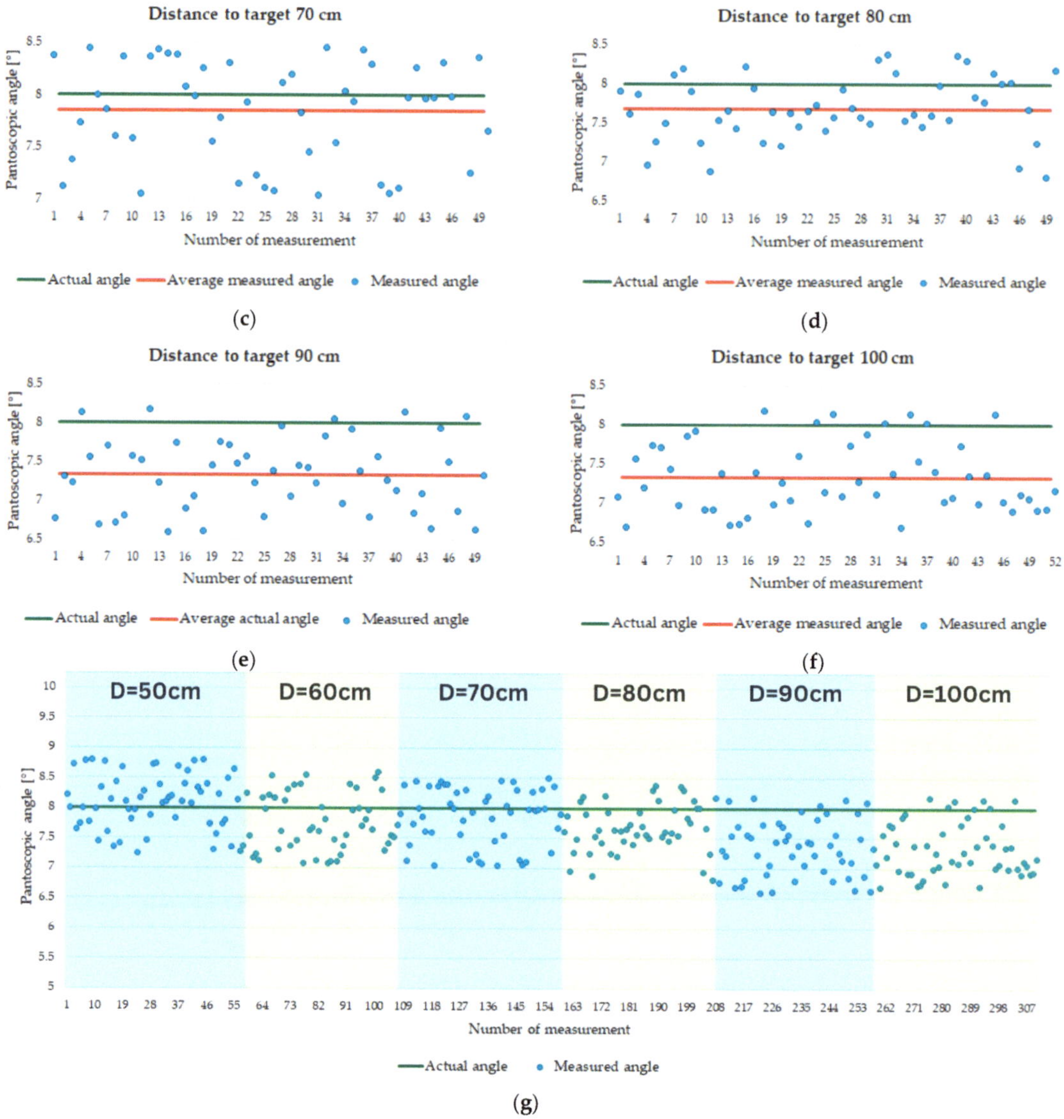

Figure 16. (**a**) Pantoscopic angle measurement at 50 cm; (**b**) Pantoscopic angle measurement at 60 cm; (**c**) Pantoscopic angle measurement at 70 cm; (**d**) Pantoscopic angle measurement at 80 cm; (**e**) Pantoscopic angle measurement at 90 cm; (**f**) Pantoscopic angle measurement at 100 cm; (**g**) Comparison chart of error distribution obtained for pantoscopic angle.

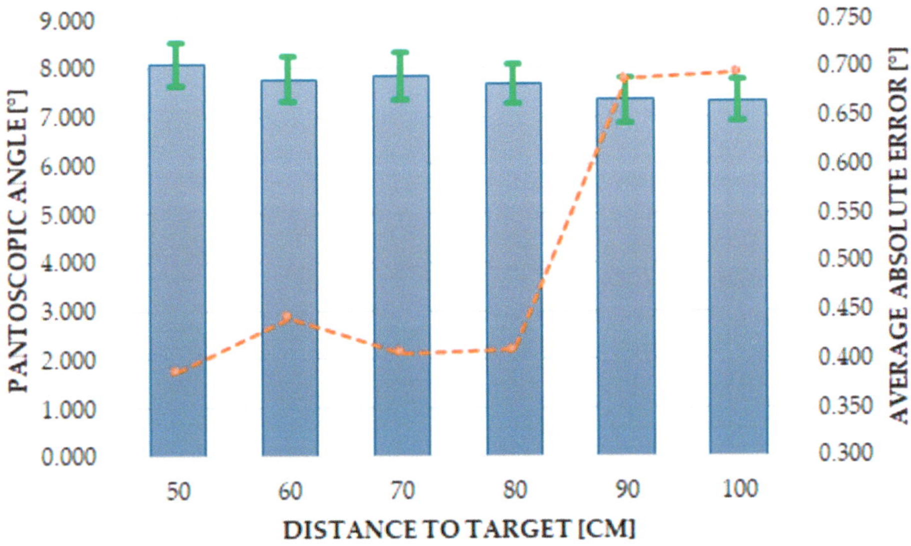

Figure 17. Comparative analysis of obtained results regarding the pantoscopic angle measurements.

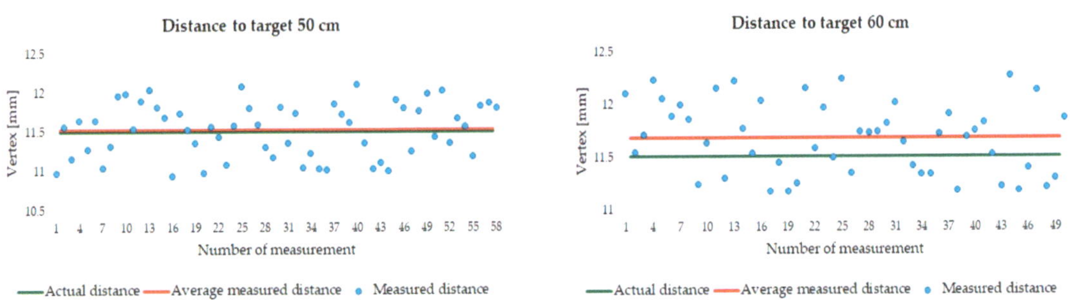

(a) (b)

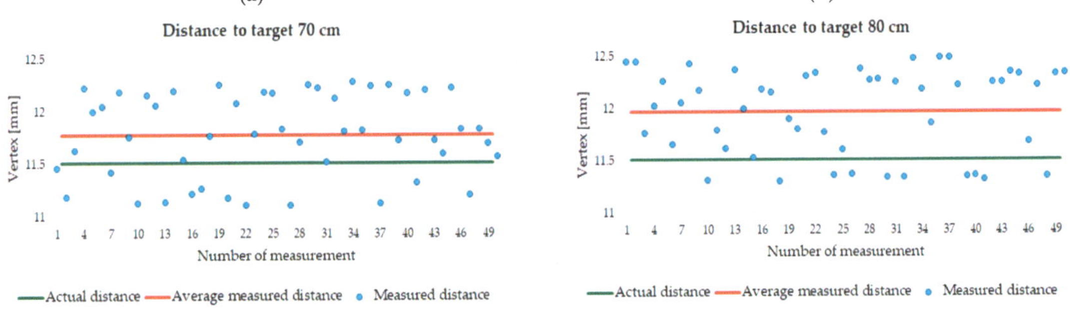

(c) (d)

Figure 18. *Cont.*

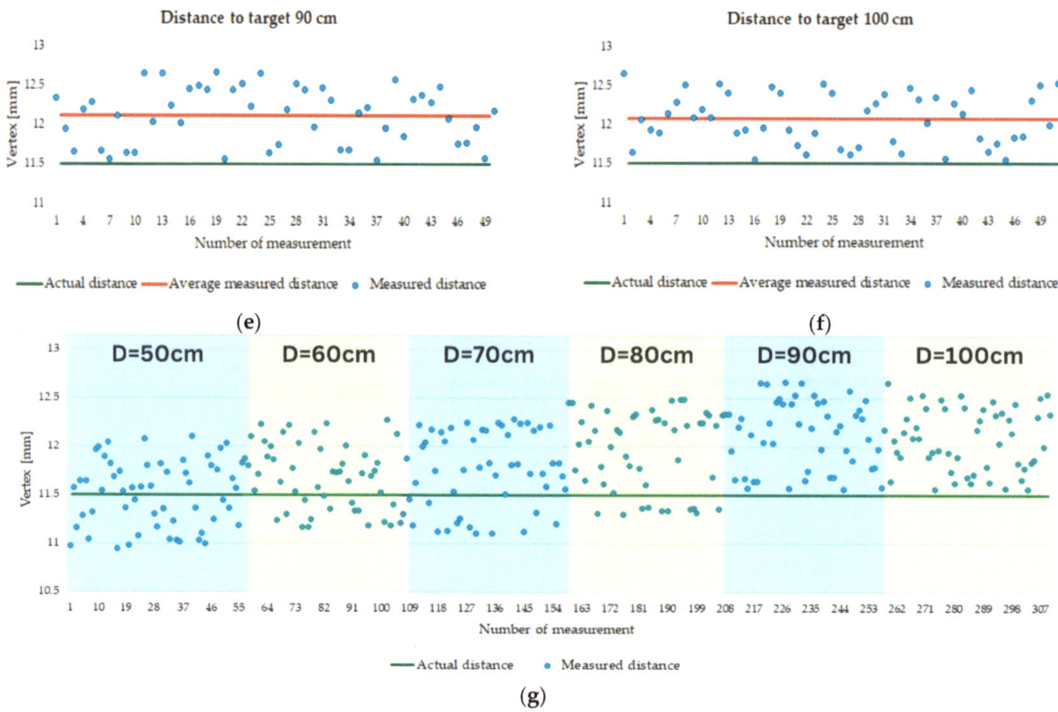

Figure 18. (**a**) Interpupillary measurement at 50 cm; (**b**) Interpupillary measurement at 60 cm; (**c**) Interpupillary measurement at 70 cm; (**d**) Interpupillary measurement at 80 cm; (**e**) Interpupillary measurement at 90 cm; (**f**) Interpupillary measurement at 100 cm; (**g**) Comparison chart of error distribution obtained for vertex distance.

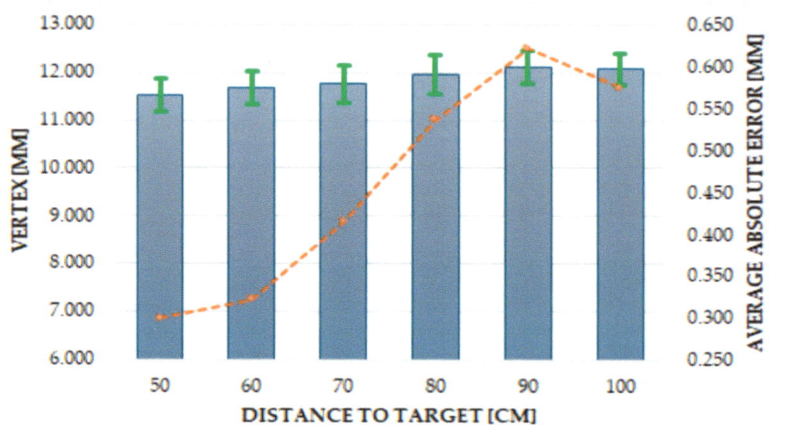

Figure 19. Comparative analysis of obtained results regarding the vertex distance measurements.

Table 5. Obtained data for pantoscopic angle measurements.

Distance to Target [cm]	Actual Angle [°]	Average Measured Angle ± SD [°]	Average Absolute Error [°]	Maximum Value [°]	Minimum Value [°]
50	8	8.084 ± 0.461	0.387	8.79	7.24
60		7.767 ± 0.467	0.443	8.60	7.07
70		7.853 ± 0.485	0.406	8.51	7.04
80		7.686 ± 0.396	0.409	8.38	6.81
90		7.336 ± 0.465	0.689	8.18	6.60
100		7.333 ± 0.443	0.695	8.18	6.69

Table 6. Obtained data for vertex distance measurements.

Distance to Target [cm]	Actual Distance [mm]	Average Measured Distance ± SD [mm]	Average Absolute Error [mm]	Maximum Value [mm]	Minimum Value [mm]
50	11.5	11.519 ± 0.342	0.298	12.10	10.94
60		11.680 ± 0.339	0.320	12.27	11.17
70		11.766 ± 0.399	0.414	12.28	11.10
80		11.965 ± 0.409	0.537	12.49	11.30
90		12.122 ± 0.353	0.622	12.67	11.56
100		12.075 ± 0.324	0.575	12.66	11.56

5. Conclusions

In the field of optometry, there is a constant demand for more precise and user-friendly equipment that enhances the customization of lenses. This paper presents a system designed to meet this need, addressing both hardware implementation and software used for processing. Previous research has detailed the development of a compliant mechanism created through additive manufacturing, which supports color markers to determine the position of glass frames relative to the patient's eyes.

A software application featuring a measurement module, whose usage and results are highlighted in this paper, was developed. This module captures and processes images, automatically detecting color markers and facial features, particularly the pupils. Using this data, an algorithm embedded in the application (not detailed in this paper) provides measurements crucial for lens customization: interpupillary distance, pantoscopic angle, vertex distance, and other parameters necessary for fitting the lens template to the user's frames.

The authors have also developed a mechatronic test bench and a methodology for testing the proposed system, comparing the application's results with real-world values. This setup ensures that external disturbances minimally impact the measurement results.

Analyzing the graphs shown in the paper, it is clearly seen how the measured average interpupillary distance increases and departs from reality as the distance to the target increases. The same general tendency can be observed in the case of average absolute errors and standard deviations. Therefore, a standard distance needs to be imposed during measurements, or a compensation mechanism needs to be implemented on the software side in order to allow for measurements to be taken from different distances.

The data obtained were interpreted graphically for individual target distances and combined to compare result dispersion across all target distances. Average measured distance, average absolute error, and standard deviations for all relevant parameters were calculated and displayed in both graphic and tabular forms.

The data, saved in an online database and later processed, showed significant differences based on the distance from the mannequin. Absolute errors for interpupillary distance increased from an average of 0.5 mm to over 2 mm. Detailed error analysis for each distance is presented in the paper figures, depicting actual distances and average measured distances with line plots and data points.

A general trend chart demonstrated a clear increase in errors beyond 70 cm, with errors rising as the mannequin's distance from the tablet increased. The absolute errors at each distance were likely due to camera movement by the optometrist during image acquisition or errors in image recognition (color and pupillary markers).

Using the current results as a starting point, further work will be conducted to prepare the system for real-life testing. Efforts are currently being made to introduce the system in a number of optometrist's offices, where, with the help of qualified professionals, a first set of information will be used to perfect the system further.

Author Contributions: Conceptualization, V.C. and E.M.; methodology, D.C., B.G. and V.C.; software, V.C. and A.C.; validation, A.C. and D.C.; formal analysis, B.G. and E.M.; investigation, V.C., E.M., and D.B.; resources; data curation, V.C.; writing—original draft preparation, E.M. and V.C.; writing—review and editing, A.C., D.C. and D.B.; visualization, V.C. and E.M.; supervision, E.M., V.C. and B.G.; project administration, V.C.; funding acquisition, V.C. All authors have read and agreed to the published version of the manuscript.

Funding: This research received no external funding.

Institutional Review Board Statement: Not applicable.

Informed Consent Statement: Not applicable.

Data Availability Statement: Data are contained within the article.

Conflicts of Interest: The authors declare no conflicts of interest.

References

1. Constantin, V.; Besnea, D.; Gramescu, B.; Moraru, E. Aspects Related to the Design and Manufacturing of an Original and Innovative Marker Support System for Use in Clinical Optometry. *Appl. Sci.* **2023**, *13*, 2859. [CrossRef]
2. Constantin, V.; Comeagă, D.; Grămescu, B.; Besnea, D.; Moraru, E. The Design and Testing of an Additive Manufacturing-Obtained Compliant Mechanism for the Complex Personalisation of Lenses in Clinical Optometry. *Appl. Sci.* **2023**, *13*, 13010. [CrossRef]
3. Pascu, A.T.; Bacescu, D.; Micu, C.A. Checking the corrective lenses for the spherical diopters hypothesis and preparing the approach for the aspherical diopters hypothesis. *U. P. B. Sci. Bull. Ser. D* **2016**, *78*, 119–130.
4. Berglund, G.; Wisniowiecki, A.; Gawedzinski, J.; Applegate, B.; Tkaczyk, T.S. Additive manufacturing for the development of optical/photonic systems and components. *Optica* **2022**, *9*, 623–638. [CrossRef]
5. Ayyildiz, O. Customised spectacles using 3-D printing technology. *Clin. Exp. Optom.* **2018**, *101*, 747–751. [CrossRef] [PubMed]
6. Tsegay, F.; Ghannam, R.; Daniel, N.; Butt, H. 3D Printing Smart Eyeglass Frames: A Review. *ACS Appl. Eng. Mater.* **2023**, *1*, 1142–1163. [CrossRef]
7. Lee, L.; Burnett, A.M.; Panos, J.G.; Paudel, P.; Keys, D.; Ansari, H.M.; Yu, M. 3-D printed spectacles: Potential, challenges and the future. *Clin. Exp. Optom.* **2020**, *103*, 590–596. [CrossRef] [PubMed]
8. Rooney, L.M.; Christopher, J.; Watson, B.; Kumar, Y.S.; Copeland, L.; Walker, L.D.; Foylan, S.; Amos, W.B.; Bauer, R.; McConnell, G. Printing, Characterizing, and Assessing Transparent 3D Printed Lenses for Optical Imaging. *Adv. Mater. Technol.* **2023**, 2400043. [CrossRef]
9. Gao, H.; An, J.; Chua, C.K.; Bourell, D.; Kuo, C.N.; Tan, D.T. 3D printed optics and photonics: Processes, materials and applications. *Mater. Today* **2023**, *69*, 107–132. [CrossRef]
10. Wang, Y.; Wang, J.; Ji, Z.; Yan, W.; Zhao, H.; Huang, W.; Liu, H. Application of bioprinting in ophthalmology. *Int. J. Bioprint.* **2022**, *8*, 552. [CrossRef] [PubMed]
11. Ruiz-Alonso, S.; Villate-Beitia, I.; Gallego, I.; Lafuente-Merchan, M.; Puras, G.; Saenz-del-Burgo, L.; Pedraz, J.L. Current insights into 3D bioprinting: An advanced approach for eye tissue regeneration. *Pharmaceutics* **2021**, *13*, 308. [CrossRef] [PubMed]
12. Kopycinska-Müller, M.; Schreiber, L.; Schwarzer-Fischer, E.; Günther, A.; Phillips, C.; Moritz, T.; Opitz, J.; Choi, Y.J.; Yun, H.S. Signal-Decay Based Approach for Visualization of Buried Defects in 3-D Printed Ceramic Components Imaged with Help of Optical Coherence Tomography. *Materials* **2023**, *16*, 3607. [CrossRef] [PubMed]
13. Wu, K.Y.; Tabari, A.; Mazerolle, É.; Tran, S.D. Towards Precision Ophthalmology: The Role of 3D Printing and Bioprinting in Oculoplastic Surgery, Retinal, Corneal, and Glaucoma Treatment. *Biomimetics* **2024**, *9*, 145. [CrossRef] [PubMed]

14. Velázquez, J.S.; Cavas, F.; Bolarín, J.M.; Alió, J.L. 3D printed personalized corneal models as a tool for improving patient's knowledge of an asymmetric disease. *Symmetry* **2020**, *12*, 151. [CrossRef]
15. Pugalendhi, A.; Ranganathan, R. A review of additive manufacturing applications in ophthalmology. *Proc. Inst. Mech. Eng. H* **2021**, *235*, 1146–1162. [CrossRef] [PubMed]

applied sciences

MDPI

Article

Combining BioTRIZ and Multi-Factor Coupling for Bionic Mechatronic System Design

Bingxin Wang * and Dehong Yu

School of Mechanical Engineering, Xi'an Jiaotong University, No.28 Xianning West Road, Xi'an 710049, China; dhyu@mail.xjtu.edu.cn

* Correspondence: wang.bx@stu.xjtu.edu.cn

Abstract: To realize the design process of bionic mechatronic systems, involving mapping from engineering to biology and inversion from biology to engineering, a novel design paradigm is introduced that integrates BioTRIZ with multi-factor coupling bionics. In the mapping stage from engineering to biology, BioTRIZ is employed to frame the concrete engineering issue as a general conflicting problem. The biological solution is refined by amalgamating the BioTRIZ solution derived from the contradiction matrix with biological instances. In the inversion stage of biology to engineering, a novel approach is proposed for constructing a bionic multi-factor coupling model, drawing inspiration from the establishment of biological multi-factor coupling model. This allows for a seamless correspondence between biological elements, such as morphology and behavior, and their respective engineering counterparts, including structure and algorithms. This correspondence ultimately achieves the engineering conceptual model that is rooted in biological principles. The practical application of this methodology is exemplified through a multi-biometric fusion bionic active vision system, underscoring its feasibility and efficacy.

Keywords: bio-inspired design; relationship mapping inversion; BioTRIZ; multi-factor coupling bionics; mechatronic system

1. Introduction

To adapt to changes in climate, habitat, and food sources, creatures have undergone diverse morphological, structural, and functional evolutions through "natural selection", enabling them to thrive in their respective environments. These adaptations have garnered significant interest not only from biologists but also from engineers seeking to harness this biodiversity through bionic principles [1–6].

Problem-driven biomimetic approaches aim to discover solutions in the biological realm for specific engineering issues. Nevertheless, evolution often reflects compromises among multiple survival necessities. For instance, the evolution of the finch beak balances various functions, such as singing, attracting mates, and grooming, rendering its structure not necessarily optimal solely for grinding food [7]. When applied to enhance the pulverizing efficiency of a jackhammer, the outcome is not an optimal but a feasible solution. On the other hand, solution-driven biomimetic approaches necessitate extracting relevant knowledge from extensive studies of living organisms to create or enhance artificial products [8,9]. However, in the context of mechatronic systems, which integrate structures, drivers, control algorithms, and more, abstracting biological knowledge into a singular mathematical, physical, or structural model not only falls short of fully describing the system overall functionality but also struggles to represent the relationships between its engineering modules.

The design of a bionic mechatronic system necessitates the realization of a comprehensive process that involves an engineering-to-biology mapping and biology-to-engineering inversion. To this end, we introduce a bio-inspired design paradigm that integrates

BioTRIZ [10] with the Extensive Model of Multi-factor Coupling Bionics (EM-MCB) [11,12]. This paradigm is based on relationship mapping inversion. We employ bionic active vision system as a representative example to illustrate the design framework of the bionic mechatronic system, which is depicted in Figure 1.

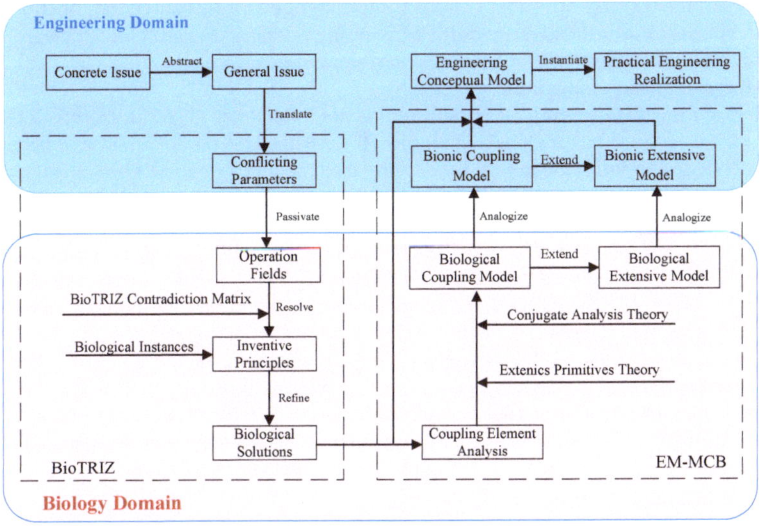

Figure 1. Bio-inspired design framework. The engineering issue is mapped onto the bio-space using BioTRIZ. Once the BioTRIZ solution and relevant biological instances are identified, the EM-MCB is constructed by examining the coupling elements that impact the biological function. Subsequently, the biological solution is translated back into the engineering domain to derive the engineering conceptual model.

In the mapping stage from engineering to biology, the engineering issue is first abstracted into a BioTRIZ conflicting problem. Through the contradiction matrix, the BioTRIZ solution is obtained. It is then combined with multiple prototypes from biological database to form a complete biological solution. This combination enables the analysis of common features and evolutionary trends observed in various creatures, and allows for a systematic analysis of the engineering requirements and a widened search range of biological instances.

In the inversion stage of biology to engineering, in order to correspond the morphological and behavioral elements of the biological system with the structure, algorithm, and other modules of the mechatronic system, a biological coupling model and an extensive model are established based on the principle of multi-factor coupling bionics. By establishing the bionic coupling model and extensive model analogously, a correspondence with the biological models is formed at the coupling element level, which in turn converts the biological solution into an engineering conceptual model.

2. Related Works

Both problem-driven and solution-driven approaches in bio-inspired design necessitate bridging the gaps between disciplines through knowledge cross-domain mapping. Vincent et al. [10] proposed BioTRIZ, which integrates classical TRIZ theory with bionic principles, to establish a "bridge" between engineering and biology. Snell-Rood et al. [13] expanded the search scope for biologically inspired solutions by transforming engineering issues into biological ones based on the concept of "functionality". Bian et al. [14] leveraged the pre-trained BERT model [15] to assess the semantic similarity between engineering and biological terms, facilitating bionic inference. Deng et al. [16] proposed a human–machine collaborative deep generative model for bionic design, visually depicting potential mappings between biomorphic forms and product shapes. Kruiper et al. [17] developed the Focused Open Biology Information Extraction (FOBIE) dataset, which is aimed at discovering relevant cross-domain scientific literature for bionics research. Numerous other scholars [18–23] have also contributed various computer-aided tools that rely on functional similarity to perform the crucial cross-domain mapping of knowledge in bionic design.

The fundamental objective of bionics is to harness insights from biological instances to tackle engineering issues, and a thorough understanding of biological prototypes serves as the foundation for achieving this. In pursuit of this goal, Ren et al. [11,12] introduced the Extensive Model of Multi-factor Coupling Bionics (EM-MCB). This model offers an efficient tool for engineering biomimetic design by delving into the mechanisms of biological prototypes and elucidating the principles of biological coupling. Nagel et al. [24] developed AskNature, an online database that employs functional representation and abstraction techniques to identify and access biological prototypes. Abdala et al. [25] created a knowledge base focused on biological effects grounded in TRIZ principles. Liu et al. [26] evaluated and selected biological prototypes based on topological, role, strategic, and structural similarity. Mak et al. [27] proposed a hierarchical approach that organizes biological phenomena into form, behavior, and principle. This structure presents a latent analogy that can inspire design solutions. Cao et al. [28] suggested abstracting biological prototypes based on their function, behavior, and structure. They further evaluated the fitness of these prototypes for engineering applications using a fuzzy triangular numbers-based algorithm. Hou et al. [29] designed a knowledge base focused on multi-biological effects and integrated TRIZ to establish a design process model by combining product functions. Bai et al. [30] combined BioTRIZ with biological coupling analysis, orthogonal analysis, and scheme merit value calculation to construct a multi-biological prototype bionic model.

In brief, bionics research has frequently focused on particular links within the biomimetic chain. Scholars endeavor to refine tools and bridge disciplinary divides, rather than address the entirety of the complex process. Much of these works have revolved around single-factor bionics. With the focus gradually shifting towards multi-factor bionics, this paper aims to combine methodology and practical application to explain the bio-inspired design paradigm, and use a typical mechatronic system to elucidate this multi-factor bio-inspired design framework more clearly.

3. Engineering-to-Biology Mapping

3.1. Problem Description

Vision, as a crucial avenue for humans and numerous vertebrates to gather environmental information, has garnered extensive research in biology [31–35]. In an effort to endow robots with comparable perceptual abilities, bionic active vision systems have become a significant focus of interest in recent years [36,37].

"Eyes in the front, the animal hunts. Eyes on the side, the animal hides" encapsulates the inherent trade-off between a wide vision field and precise visual localization in nature. Predators, with their powerful stereoscopic vision, can pinpoint the exact location of their prey, but may sacrifice a comprehensive awareness of their surroundings. Conversely, prey animals possess a broad vision field that allows them to detect potential predators in their environment, but this comes at the cost of developing binocular stereo vision, making precise localization nearly impossible.

The majority of existing bionic active vision systems adopt a binocular structure, and are utilized for environmental monitoring, situational awareness, object detection, and tracking, among other applications [38–41]. These systems typically emulate the visual system of a specific vertebrate [42–44], either by modeling binocular stereo vision for 3D measurements or by replicating a wide vision field for environmental monitoring and scene comprehension. Additionally, there are visual systems that enable switching between these two functions through mimicking eye movements, offering a compromise between the two, but they cannot simultaneously acquire both global vision and precise information [45].

The application environment of machine vision is increasingly unstructured and complex. Our objective is to devise a bionic vision system that can simultaneously maintain a global vision field and acquire accurate local information. To achieve this, we incorporate a bio-inspired design paradigm that implements engineering-to-biology mapping and biology-to-engineering inversion during the design process.

3.2. BioTRIZ

Engineering-to-biology mapping is essentially a cross-domain knowledge translation. Through numerous patent analysis, TRIZ [46] has revealed that every creative patent is essentially solving a conflicting problem, and that the basic principles for addressing these contradictions are highly reusable.

Possessing a wide vision field and acquiring precise information often present a conflicting pair: an improvement in one aspect typically leads to a deterioration in the other. In this context, the application of TRIZ becomes a viable solution. Notably, TRIZ is a systematic theory that emerges from the refinement and reorganization of existing knowledge across diverse fields [47]. Its strength lies in the ability to address problems in various domains using common principles, facilitating the knowledge transfer from one field to another. This aligns well with the fundamental requirements of bio-inspired design, which aims to translate functions, structures, and principles across different domains [48].

TRIZ has distilled 39 widely applicable Engineering Parameters (EPs) from numerous patents and introduced 40 universally relevant Inventive Principles (IPs). These IPs are grounded in the common "technical contradiction" where one parameter improves while another deteriorates. However, TRIZ originated in the field of things artificial, non-living, technical, and engineering. To integrate TRIZ with the biology domain and cater to the demands of bionics, Vincent et al. proposed BioTRIZ [10]. BioTRIZ replaces the 39 EPs with 6 Operational Fields (OFs): *substance*, *structure*, *space*, *time*, *energy*, and *information*. Furthermore, it established the BioTRIZ contradiction matrix, as presented in Table 1. This shift to OFs not only condenses the original EPs and IPs of TRIZ, but also simplifies and streamlines the invention process, making it more logical and accessible.

Table 1. BioTRIZ contradiction matrix [10]. Select one OF that needs to be improved from the six arranged vertically, and then identify the OF that will be deteriorative from the six listed horizontally. The intersection of the selected row and column will indicate the corresponding IPs, which constitutes the BioTRIZ solution.

Fields	Substance	Structure	Space	Time	Energy	Information
Substance	13 15 17 20 31 40	1–3 15 24 26	1 5 13 15 31	15 19 27 29 30	3 6 9 25 31 35	3 25 26
Structure	1 10 15 19	1 15 19 24 34	10	1 2 4	1 2 4	1 3 4 15 19 24 25 35
Space	3 14 15 25	2–5 10 15 19	4 5 36 14 17	1 19 29	1 3 4 15 19	3 15 21 24
Time	1 3 15 20 25 38	1–4 6 15 17 19	1–4 7 38	2 3 11 20 26	3 9 15 20 22 25	1–3 10 19 23
Energy	1 3 13 14 17 25 31	1 3 5 6 25 36 40	1 3 4 15 25	3 10 23 25 35	3 5 9 22 25 32 37	1 3 4 15 16 25
Information	1 6 22	1 3 6 18 22 24 32 34 40	3 20 22 25 33	2 3 9 17 22	1 3 6 22 32	3 10 16 23 25

We apply BioTRIZ in the mapping stage from engineering to biology, as illustrated in Figure 2. Initially, the engineering issue is formulated as a BioTRIZ conflicting pair. Subsequently, a BioTRIZ solution is retrieved from the contradiction matrix. Ultimately, this solution is integrated with biological instances to derive a complete biological solution.

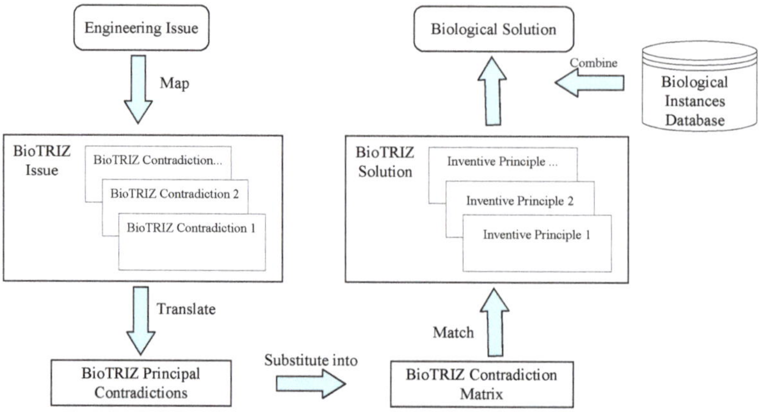

Figure 2. BioTRIZ implementation. When tackling an invention problem with BioTRIZ, the initial step involves modeling the engineering issue as a BioTRIZ issue, utilizing OFs to articulate the conflicts. Subsequently, IPs that align with the requirements are acquired by referencing the BioTRIZ contradiction matrix. Lastly, biological solutions are derived by amalgamating the IPs with prototypes present in the biological database.

3.3. BioTRIZ Solution

To resolve the problem presented in Section 3.1, the engineering contradiction between achieving a wide vision field and precise information acquisition is initially converted into a BioTRIZ contradiction.

The parameters related to the vision field in a bionic binocular vision system typically encompass factors such as the viewing angle of image sensors and the direction of optical axis related to the system midline, as illustrated in Figure 3. The image captured by cameras encompasses a three-dimensional space. If the sensor is mounted on a gimbal, it can be regarded as a moving object; otherwise, it is considered a stationary object. Consequently, the issues pertaining to the vision field can be framed as

- EP7 *Volume of moving object*; or EP8 *Volume of stationary object*.

The direction of optical axis determines the appearance of the system, which can be abstracted as

- EP12 *Shape*.

Furthermore, a wide vision field results in a lack of precise information, and a narrow vision field leads to insufficient global information, which can be abstracted as

- EP24 *Loss of information*.

According to Appendix 2 of the literature [10], EP7, EP8, and EP12 fall under the *space* field, whereas EP24 pertains to the *information* field. Consequently, the BioTRIZ problem we aim to address is to prevent deterioration of the *information* field when optimizing the *space* field. This aligns with the observations made in biological vision system, where both predator and prey vision systems experience a loss of either global or local information. The intersection of the *space* field and the *information* field in Table 1 represents potential BioTRIZ solutions, including the following IPs:

- IP3 *Local Quality*.
    - IP3-1: Change an object's structure, action, environment, or external influence/impact from uniform to non-uniform.
    - IP3-2: Make each part of an object function in conditions most suitable for its operation.

- IP3-3: Make each part of an object fulfil a different and/or complementary useful function.

- IP15 *Dynamics*.
  - IP15-1: Change the object (or outside environment) for optimal performance at every stage of operation, make them adaptable.
  - IP15-2: Divide an object into parts capable of movement relative to each other.
  - IP15-3: Change from immobile to mobile.
  - IP15-4: Increase the degree of free motion.
- IP21 *Skipping*.
  - Conduct a process or stages of it (e.g., destructive, harmful, hazardous operations) at high speed.
- IP24 *Intermediary*.
  - IP24-1: Use an intermediary carrier article or intermediary process.
  - IP24-2: Merge one object temporarily with another.

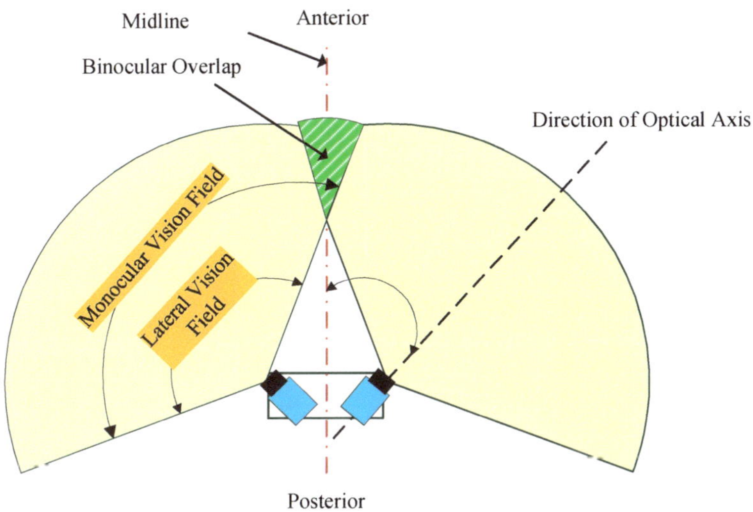

Figure 3. Illustration of the bionic binocular vision system parameters. The viewing angle of an image sensor represents the monocular vision field range. The direction of optical axis dictates the extent of binocular overlap. The overall vision field is comprised of the left and right lateral vision fields and the binocular overlap. Regions beyond these are designated as blind areas.

3.4. Biological Prototypes

Combining the IPs with biological instances can result in a complete biological solution, as presented in Table 2. We utilize strategies related to "eyes" and "vision" from the AskNature online database [24] as biological prototypes. The biological instances indicate several key evolutionary directions in solving survival problems similar to our engineering issues:

- Adding auxiliary eyes to enhance the existing capability of visual systems.
- Differentiating the functional roles of the left and right eyes, which originally served identical purposes, allowing them to independently fulfill distinct functional requirements.
- Modifying the internal structure of the eyes to enable different parts to perform specialized functions, thus increasing the versatility and efficiency of the visual system.
- Enhancing the range and speed of eye movements to achieve functional transitions between a wide vision field and local information acquisition.

Table 2. BioTRIZ solutions and biological instances. The table comprises three columns that present the results obtained in engineering-to-biology mapping, arranged from left to right. Column 1 exhibits the BioTRIZ issues (OFs), column 2 displays the BioTRIZ solutions (IPs), and column 3 illustrates the corresponding biological instances. This table serves as complete biological solution for engineering-to-biology inversion.

OFs	IPs	Supporting Biological Instances
Improved: *Space* Deteriorated: *Information*	IP3 *Local Quality* IP15 *Dynamics* IP21 *Skipping* IP24 *Intermediary*	• Six-eyed spookfish's eyes: Two pairs auxiliary, one pair primary. • Jumping spider's eyes: Eight total, two for stereoscopic vision, six for omnidirectional. • Brownsnout spookfish's auxiliary eyes: Create clear images via light reflection and focusing. • Whirligig beetle's eyes: One submerged underwater to hunt for prey, one above the water to keep watch for predators. • Starling's eyes: One for overall scene, one for details. • Anableps anableps' lens: Thicker lower part for underwater gaze, upper part for air scanning. • Nocturnal gecko's multifocal lens: Different parts of the lens focus a different range of wavelengths onto the eye's light-sensitive cells. • Scallop's retinas: One responds to light, the other to sudden darkness. • Hammerhead shark's eyes: Located on "hammer" sides, enhancing stereoscopic perception and wide view. • Ghost crab's eyes: On movable stalks, providing full range of vision. • Chameleon's eyes: Rotate freely, switching between monocular and binocular vision. • Vertebrate's reflective tapetum: Improves low-light visual sensitivity. • Horseshoe crab's eyes: Sensitive to polarized light, reducing sun glare. • Jewel scarab beetle's eyes: Distinguish polarized from unpolarized light. • Lobster's eyes: Feature square tubes focusing reflected light on retina. • West Indian wood snake's eyes: Release blood to deter predators. • Locust's eyes: Recognize only movement interfering with flight path. • Reef heron's head position: Adjusts for surface light refraction, maintaining relationship between real and apparent prey depth. • Kestrel's eyes: Four reflexes enable focus during body movement. • Dragonfly's eyes: Capture up to 300 images/second, enhancing movement perception and compensating for lack of visual sharpness.

A single biological instance often balances multiple survival needs, making it difficult to derive optimal solutions to engineering problems by mimicking a specific species. Instead, we aim to integrate various demand-fulfilling features from the above evolutionary directions to effectively address engineering issues.

4. Biology-to-Engineering Inversion

4.1. Extensive Model of Multi-Factor Coupling Bionics

After obtaining the biological instances and inventive principles, the biological solutions need to be inverted to the engineering domain, as depicted in Figure 4. In traditional single-factor bionics, engineers tend to focus on a single aspect of morphology, structure, or neural mechanism and design the bionic model or algorithm based solely on that factor. Nevertheless, the adaptive functions displayed by organisms are actually the outcome of the interplay between various related factors. Likewise, in a mechatronic system, the mechanical structure, actuator, and software must collaborate seamlessly. In this case, it is difficult to describe the interactions between these engineering modules using solely mathematical, physical, or structural model.

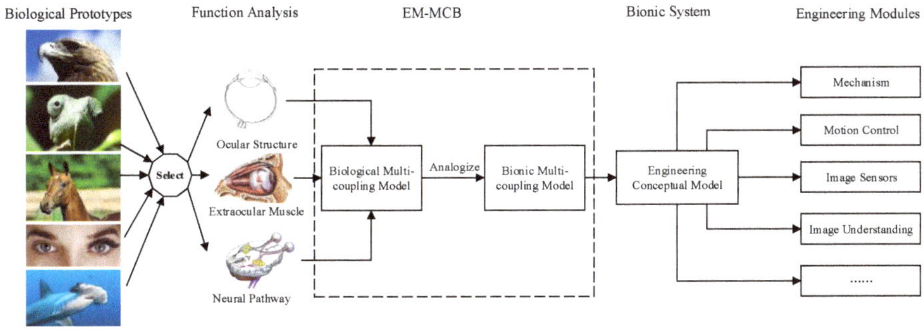

Figure 4. Biology to engineering inversion. Once a solution is derived from the biology domain, the translation of biological properties into engineering realizations becomes necessary. Initially, appropriate biological prototypes are identified as bionic targets, and their distinctive features, such as structure, morphology, and neural mechanism, are thoroughly analyzed. Subsequently, the EM-MCB is constructed using these BCEs and analogous principles in the engineering domain. Eventually, a comprehensive bionic system and an engineering conceptual model with several modules can be created.

To provide a comprehensive understanding of the biological coupling mechanism, Ren et al. introduced the Extensive Model of Multi-factor Coupling Bionics (EM-MCB) [11,12]. This model defines the diverse elements that impact biological functions as Biological Coupling Elements (BCEs) and the ways of interaction between these elements as Biological Coupling Ways (BCWs). To mirror similar coupling mechanisms in mechatronic systems, we have analogously established an EM-MCB framework in the engineering realm. Within this framework, the elements that shape system functions are designated as Engineering Coupling Elements (ECEs), while the ways of association between these modules are termed Engineering Coupling Ways (ECWs). By integrating the multi-factor coupling model of the bionic system with the biological solution, we arrive at the engineering conceptual model. Once the structure, specifications, and algorithms of this conceptual model are firmly established, it can be instantiated into engineering forms.

4.2. Biological Model

A biological model of EM-MCB comprises two primary components: a coupling model and an extensive model. The coupling model delves into the biological coupling mechanism, identifying all the coupling elements that impact the biological function. The extensive model, rooted in the theory of extenics primitives and the theory of conjugate analysis [49], treats all these coupling elements as the hard part and the relationships between them as the soft part.

To synthesize the visual advantages observed in various biological prototypes, we have established a biological coupling model that is based on the shared features of vertebrate oculomotor and ocular structures, as illustrated in Figure 5. From this model, it becomes evident that visual perception arises from the integration of multiple components, including eye layout, eyeball structure, and the optic nerve. The extraocular muscles play a crucial role in controlling eye movements such as scanning and fixating. Meanwhile, the optic nerve implements visual attention and transmits sensory stimuli to the cerebral cortex for higher-level visual processing.

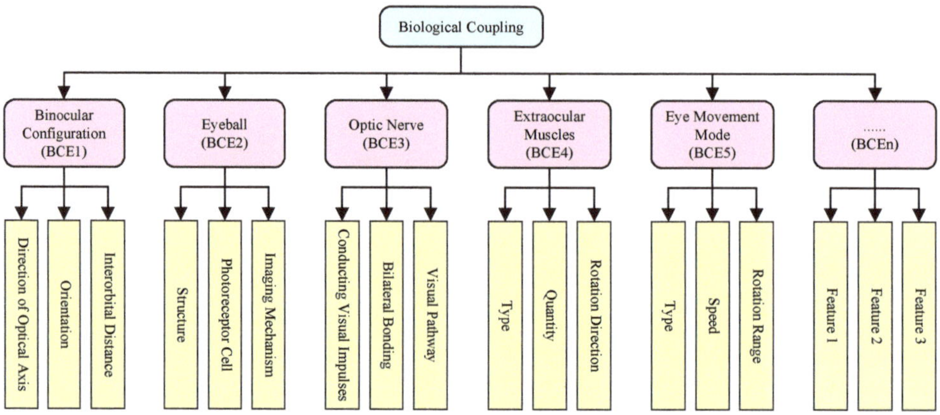

Figure 5. The Biological Coupling Model of Binocular Vision for Vertebrates. In this model, BCEs represent the factors that affect the visual perception of vertebrates. These elements encompass binocular configuration, which involves the eyes' positional relationship, head position, and orientation, as well as eyeball shape and structure. The optic nerve conducts visual signals to the cerebral cortex, forming the visual pathway, while extraocular muscles enable eye rotations for sweeping and gazing movements.

Importantly, the number of BCEs included in the model can be expanded based on the specific research objectives. Similarly, the descriptions of BCEs can be progressively refined in a hierarchical manner to meet the evolving needs of the study. This flexibility allows the model to serve as a dynamic tool for exploring and understanding the complexities of vertebrate vision.

After further analyzing BCEs and referring to the values provided in [50–60], the BCEs depicted in Figure 5 can be described as follows:

$$M_1 = \begin{bmatrix} \text{Structure} & \text{Binocular} \\ & \text{Direction of Optical Axis: } 0^\circ \sim 90^\circ \\ & \text{Complete Vision Field: } 150^\circ \sim 360^\circ \\ & \text{Binocular Overlap: } 10^\circ \sim 124^\circ \end{bmatrix} \quad (1)$$

$$M_2 = \begin{bmatrix} \text{Structure} & \text{Eyeball} \\ & \text{Vision Field: } 105^\circ \sim 190^\circ \\ & \text{Fovea Num: } 0 \sim 2 \end{bmatrix} \quad (2)$$

$$M_3 = \begin{bmatrix} \text{Material} & \text{Optic Nerve} \\ & \text{Length: } 42\text{mm} \sim 47\text{mm} \end{bmatrix} \quad (3)$$

$$M_4 = \begin{bmatrix} \text{Structure} & \text{Extraocular Muscle} \\ & \text{Num: } 6 \\ & \text{Rotation: Horz, Vert} \\ & \text{Type: Rectus, Obliques} \end{bmatrix} \quad (4)$$

$$M_5 = \begin{bmatrix} \text{Behavior} & \text{Eye Movement} \\ & \text{Range: } 1^\circ \sim 180^\circ \\ & \text{Speed: } \leq 600^\circ/\text{s} \end{bmatrix} \quad (5)$$

The BCWs can be described as follows:

$$R = \begin{bmatrix} \text{Coupling Way} & \text{Previous:} M_i \\ & \text{Next: } M_j \\ & \text{Coupling Degree: } v_3 \\ & \text{Position Relationship: } v_4 \\ & \vdots \\ & \text{Permanency: } v_m \end{bmatrix} \tag{6}$$

In this matrix, M_i and M_j represent the i-th and j-th BCE, respectively, where both i and j are integers satisfying $1 \leq i, j \leq 5$. And v_3, v_4, and v_m satisfy the following formulas:

$$\begin{aligned} v_3 &= \{\text{Compounding, fusion, compounding, chimerism, unionization, ...}\} \\ v_4 &= \{\text{Top–Bottom, Left–Right, Front–Back, Stacked, ...}\} \\ v_m &= \{\text{Permanent, temporary}\} \end{aligned}$$

The biological EM-MCB can be summarized as follows:

$$\begin{aligned} B &= M_1 \oplus M_2 \oplus M_3 \oplus M_4 \oplus M_5 \oplus R \\ &= \begin{bmatrix} \text{Biological Coupling} & \text{Function} & \text{Monitoring, hunting, hiding, etc.} \\ & \text{BCE} & M_1 \wedge M_2 \wedge M_3 \wedge M_4 \wedge M_5 \\ & \text{BCW} & R \\ & \text{Working Env} & \text{Air} \wedge \text{Water} \end{bmatrix} \end{aligned} \tag{7}$$

where $\oplus$ signifies the generalized connection between coupling elements, while $\wedge$ represents logical AND.

4.3. Bionic Model

The bionic EM-MCB aims to analogize and modify the biological EM-MCB based on engineering requirements through the application of bionics principles. This model not only embodies the principles of biological coupling but also incorporates engineering needs.

Referring to the biological model, a bionic EM-MCB also encompasses a coupling model and an extensive model. Based on the commonly accepted structure of a bionic active vision system [40–46], a coupling model for the bionic system is established, as illustrated in Figure 6. The perception of the bionic visual system is influenced by a range of factors including binocular configuration, image sensors, information transmission, and more. The motion mechanism is used to mimic the eye movements of vertebrates. Bionic algorithms are employed to accomplish visual perception tasks. These ECEs align closely with those of the biological BCEs: image sensor corresponds to eyeball, mechanism to extraocular muscles, motion control to eye movement pattern, and so on. Likewise, the ECEs in the model can be increased as the research progresses, and the description of a single ECE can be further stratified and refined according to the requirements.

Analogous to Figure 5, we have constructed the bionic coupling model tailored for engineering applications, as depicted in Figure 6. Owing to different specific applications, there exist notable variations in the implementation of sensors, algorithms, and performance metrics employed in bionic systems. In an extensive model, features must be quantitatively represented. Our objective is to introduce a general conceptual framework, so we will refrain from delving into constructing a specific extensive model.

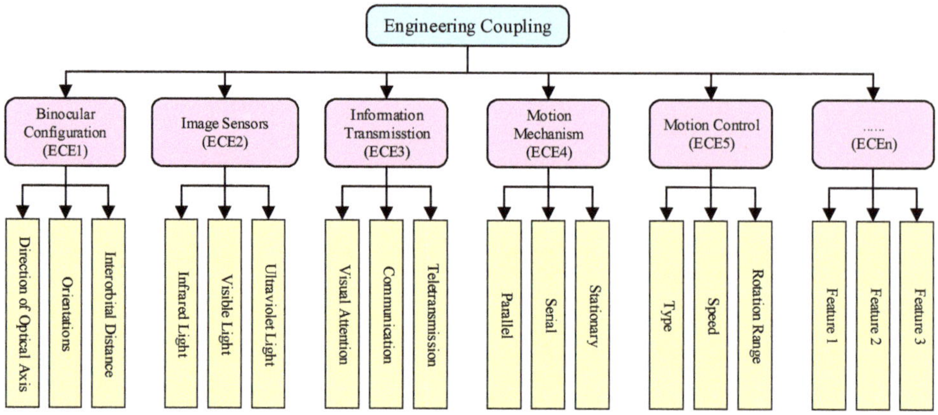

Figure 6. The coupling model of the bionic active vision system. This model encompasses several ECEs and their features. The binocular configuration involves the relative positioning of the eyes and orientations. Image sensors can be a variety of different wavelengths and vision fields. Information transmission relies on visual perception algorithms and communication with higher-level computational units. The motion mechanism enables the rotation and shifting of image sensors, while motion control achieves sweeping and gazing movements.

4.4. Engineering Conceptual Model

By combining the BioTIRZ solution, the shared characteristics of biological instances, and the bionic EM-MCB, we can ultimately derive an engineering conceptual model, as illustrated in Figure 7.

The bionic active vision system must concurrently scan the global visual field and capture local precise information. To achieve this, the following ECEs have been implemented:

- ECE1 *Binocular Configuration.*
  - Drawing inspiration from the binocular arrangement of prey animals, we have adopted a lateral layout with optical axes perpendicular to the system midline, ensuring a wide vision field.
- ECE2 *Image Sensors.*
  - Inspired by the visual enhancement observed in auxiliary eyes of jumping spiders and six-eyed ghostfish, the retinal and foveal advantages in visual information acquisition, the double foveal distribution in raptors [50,51,55,60], and recommendations from IP3-2, we have increased the number of image sensors. Wide-angle cameras O_1 and O_2 perform global searching, while narrow-angle cameras C_1, C_2, C_3, and C_4 are dedicated to capturing local details. In Figure 7, assuming random target appearance within the panoramic range, four cameras are positioned at 90° intervals, echoing the auxiliary eye count in biological instances.
- ECE3 *Information Transmission.*
  - Mimicking the optic nerve conduction and visual attention pathway [61], we process the panoramic imagery using a dynamic target recognition algorithm akin to frog or eagle vision. Recognition results then guide the narrow-angle cameras to track and acquire detailed target information.
- ECE4 *Motion Mechanism.*
  - The wide-angle cameras stay fixed. The narrow-angle cameras can be mounted on series or parallel mechanisms, drawing from the characteristics of extraocular muscles and IP3-3. The platform's degrees of freedom and angular range are tailored to practical requirements.

- ECE5 *Motion Control.*
  - Based on specific requirements, including single or multi-target tracking and 3D measurements, the gimbals equipped with narrow-angle cameras have the capability to mimic chameleon-like independent eye movements, in addition to binocular synergistic eye movements, such as scanning and gazing.

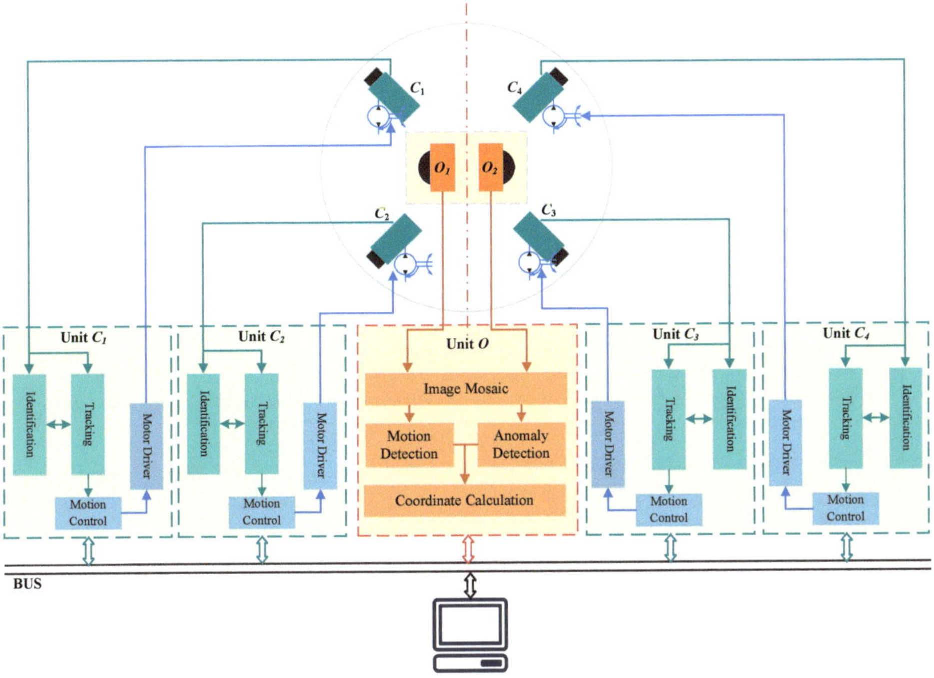

Figure 7. Engineering conceptual model of the bionic active vision system. The schematic provides a comprehensive overview of the mechatronic system structure, driver, and algorithms. It features wide-angle cameras O_1 and O_2 mounted back-to-back, offering a 360° panoramic view. This design mimics prey animals' eye structure, enabling quick object localization within the panoramic range using detection algorithms. Additionally, narrow-angle cameras C_1, C_2, C_3, and C_4 are positioned at 90° intervals and equipped with motion mechanisms for orientation changes. Once a tracking target is identified, one or two of these narrow-angle cameras are activated for tracking purposes or 3D measurement. Advanced Intelligent Decision is used to mimic the visual cortex of the brain. When considering the bionic active vision system as a perceptual module, the decision unit is capable of making high-level decisions for mechatronic systems, such as robots, through the analysis of information abstracted from the visual perception module.

5. Conclusions

This paper endeavors to introduce a novel bionic design paradigm, which integrates BioTRIZ with multi-factor coupling bionics. This methodology provides a general conceptual design framework for the bionic systems that necessitate the realization of a comprehensive process that involves engineering-to-biology mapping and biology-to-engineering inversion.

To intuitively explain the framework, the design process of a bionic vision system integrating multiple biological characteristics is presented. The design results show that this system not only draws inspiration from biological instances but also enhances the original capabilities of these living creatures. As a result, it offers a remarkable bionic solution for synchronously achieving omnidirectional surveillance, precise localization, and multi-target tracking in engineering applications.

Our future research will be directed towards refining this general framework to more precisely align with the design imperatives of specific engineering challenges. Additionally, we will concentrate on the concrete implementation strategies for the engineering conceptual model of the bionic active vision system designed in this study, meticulously selecting appropriate mechanical structures and equipment models to facilitate the acquisition of more quantifiable performance metrics.

Author Contributions: Formal analysis, B.W.; Methodology, B.W.; Project administration, D.Y.; Supervision, D.Y.; Writing—original draft, B.W.; Writing—review and editing, D.Y. All authors have read and agreed to the published version of the manuscript.

Funding: This research was funded by the National Natural Science Foundation of China under Grant No. 51375368.

Data Availability Statement: The original contributions presented in the study are included in the article, further inquiries can be directed to the corresponding author.

Conflicts of Interest: The paper is original in its contents and is not under consideration for publication in any other journals or proceedings. On behalf of all authors, the corresponding author states that there are no competing financial interests or personal relationships that could have appeared to influence the work reported in this paper. The funders had no role in the design of the study; in the collection, analyses, or interpretation of data; in the writing of the manuscript; or in the decision to publish the results.

References

1. Cheong, H.; Shu, L. Using templates and mapping strategies to support analogical transfer in biomimetic design. *Des. Stud.* **2013**, *34*, 706–728. [CrossRef]
2. Helms, M.; Vattam, S.S.; Goel, A.K. Biologically inspired design: Process and products. *Des. Stud.* **2009**, *30*, 606–622. [CrossRef]
3. Mak, T.; Shu, L. Using descriptions of biological phenomena for idea generation. *Res. Eng. Des.* **2008**, *19*, 21–28. [CrossRef]
4. Benyus, J.M. *Biomimicry: Innovation Inspired by Nature*; Harper Perennial: New York, NY, USA, 1997.
5. Nagel, R.L.; Midha, P.A.; Tinsley, A.; Stone, R.B.; McAdams, D.A.; Shu, L. Exploring the use of functional models in biomimetic conceptual design. *J. Mech. Des.* **2008**, *130*, 121102. [CrossRef]
6. Hoyos, C.M.; Fiorentino, C. Bio-utilization. *Int. J. Des. Objects* **2017**, *10*, 1.
7. Snell-Rood, E.C.; Smirnoff, D. Biology for biomimetics I: Function as an interdisciplinary bridge in bio-inspired design. *Bioinspir Biomimetics* **2023**, *18*, 052001. [CrossRef]
8. Nkandu, M.I.; Alibaba, H.Z. Biomimicry as an alternative approach to sustainability. *Archit. Res.* **2018**, *8*, 1–11.
9. Dash, S.P. Application of biomimicry in building design. *Int. J. Civ. Eng. Technol.* **2018**, *9*, 644–660.
10. Vincent, J.F.; Bogatyreva, O.A.; Bogatyrev, N.R.; Bowyer, A.; Pahl, A.K. Biomimetics: Its practice and theory. *J. R. Soc. Interface* **2006**, *3*, 471–482. [CrossRef]
11. Ren, L.; Liang, Y. Biological couplings: Classification and characteristic rules. *Sci. China Ser. Technol. Sci.* **2009**, *52*, 2791–2800. [CrossRef]
12. Ren, L.; Liang, Y. Biological couplings: Function, characteristics and implementation mode. *Sci. China Technol. Sci.* **2010**, *53*, 379–387. [CrossRef]
13. Snell-Rood, E. Interdisciplinarity: Bring biologists into biomimetics. *Nature* **2016**, *529*, 277–278. [CrossRef]
14. Bian, Z.; Luo, S.; Zheng, F.; Wang, L.; Shan, P. Semantic reasoning of product biologically inspired design based on BERT. *Appl Sci.* **2021**, *11*, 12082. [CrossRef]
15. Devlin, J.; Chang, M.W.; Lee, K.; Toutanova, K. Bert: Pre-training of deep bidirectional transformers for language understanding. *arXiv* **2018**, arXiv:1810.04805. https://doi.org/10.48550/arXiv.1810.04805.
16. Deng, Z.; Lv, J.; Liu, X.; Hou, Y. Bionic Design Model for Co-creative Product Innovation Based on Deep Generative and BID. *Int J. Comput. Intell. Syst.* **2023**, *16*, 8. [CrossRef]
17. Kruiper, R.; Vincent, J.F.; Chen-Burger, J.; Desmulliez, M.P.; Konstas, I. A scientific information extraction dataset for nature inspired engineering. *arXiv* **2020**, arXiv:2005.07753.
18. Vandevenne, D.; Verhaegen, P.A.; Dewulf, S.; Duflou, J.R. A scalable approach for ideation in biologically inspired design. *AI EDAM* **2015**, *29*, 19–31. [CrossRef]
19. Vandevenne, D.; Pieters, T.; Duflou, J.R. Enhancing novelty with knowledge-based support for Biologically-Inspired Design. *Des Stud.* **2016**, *46*, 152–173. [CrossRef]
20. Shu, L.; Cheong, H. A Natural Language Approach to Biomimetic Design In *Biologically Inspired Design: Computational Methods and Tools*; Springer: London, UK, 2014; pp. 29–61, ISBN 978-1-4471-5248-4 [CrossRef]

21. Cheong, H.; Shu, L. Retrieving causally related functions from natural-language text for biomimetic design. *J. Mech. Des.* **2014**, *136*, 081008. [CrossRef]
22. Rugaber, S.; Bhati, S.; Goswami, V.; Spiliopoulou, E.; Azad, S.; Koushik, S.; Kulkarni, R.; Kumble, M.; Sarathy, S.; Goel, A. Knowledge extraction and annotation for cross-domain textual case-based reasoning in biologically inspired design. In Proceedings of the Case-Based Reasoning Research and Development: 24th International Conference, ICCBR 2016, Atlanta, GA, USA, 31 October–2 November 2016; Proceedings 24; Springer: Berlin/Heidelberg, Germany, 2016; pp. 342–355. [CrossRef]
23. Zhao, Y.; Baldini, I.; Sattigeri, P.; Padhi, I.; Lee, Y.K.; Smith, E. Data driven techniques for organizing scientific articles relevant to biomimicry. In Proceedings of the 2018 AAAI/ACM Conference on AI, Ethics, and Society, New Orleans, LA, USA, 2–3 February 2018; pp. 347–353. [CrossRef]
24. Nagel, J.K.; Nagel, R.L.; Stone, R.B.; McAdams, D.A. Function-based, biologically inspired concept generation. *Ai Edam* **2010**, *24*, 521–535. [CrossRef]
25. Abdala, L.N.; Fernandes, R.B.; Ogliari, A.; Löwer, M.; Feldhusen, J. Creative contributions of the methods of inventive principles of TRIZ and BioTRIZ to problem solving. *J. Mech. Des.* **2017**, *139*, 082001. [CrossRef]
26. Liu, X.; Li, J.; Chen, L.; Cheng, G. Bionic prototype acquisition incorporating extension and multi-level knowledge modeling. *J. Mech. Eng.* **2019**, *55*, 150–160.
27. Mak, T.; Shu, L. Abstraction of biological analogies for design. *Cirp Ann.* **2004**, *53*, 117–120. [CrossRef]
28. Cao, G.; Sun, Y.; Tan, R.; Zhang, J.; Liu, W. A function-oriented biologically analogical approach for constructing the design concept of smart product in Industry 4.0. *Adv. Eng. Inform.* **2021**, *49*, 101352. [CrossRef]
29. Hou, X.T.; Liu, W.; Cao, G.Z.; Wu, Z.f.; Guo, Z.B. Research on design method of function combination product based on multi biological effects. *Chin. J. Eng. Des.* **2017**, *24*, 18–26.
30. Bai, Z.; Song, M.; Zhang, X.; Zhang, J. Biological Prototype Acquisition Based on Biological Coupling in Bionic Design. *Appl. Bionics Biomech.* **2022**, *2022*, 8458243. [CrossRef]
31. Heesy, C.P. Seeing in stereo: The ecology and evolution of primate binocular vision and stereopsis. *Evol. Anthropol. Issues News Rev.* **2009**, *18*, 21–35. [CrossRef]
32. Read, J.C. Binocular vision and stereopsis across the animal kingdom. *Annu. Rev. Vis. Sci.* **2021**, *7*, 389–415. [CrossRef]
33. Tyrrell, L.P.; Fernández-Juricic, E. Avian binocular vision: It's not just about what birds can see, it's also about what they can't. *PLoS ONE* **2017**, *12*, e0173235. [CrossRef]
34. Potier, S.; Mitkus, M.; Kelber, A. Visual adaptations of diurnal and nocturnal raptors. In *Seminars in Cell & Developmental Biology*; Elsevier: London, UK, 2020; Volume 106, pp. 116–126. [CrossRef]
35. Nilsson, D.E. The diversity of eyes and vision. *Annu. Rev. Vis. Sci.* **2021**, *7*, 19–41. [CrossRef]
36. Zhang, H.; Lee, S. Robot bionic vision technologies: A review. *Appl. Sci.* **2022**, *12*, 7970. [CrossRef]
37. Zhai, G.; Zhang, W.; Hu, W.; Ji, Z. Coal mine rescue robots based on binocular vision: A review of the state of the art. *IEEE Access* **2020**, *8*, 130561–130575. [CrossRef]
38. Zhang, S.; Li, B.; Ren, F.; Dong, R. High-precision measurement of binocular telecentric vision system with novel calibration and matching methods. *IEEE Access* **2019**, *7*, 54682–54692. [CrossRef]
39. Liu, Y.; Zhu, D.; Peng, J.; Wang, X.; Wang, L.; Chen, L.; Li, J.; Zhang, X. Real-time robust stereo visual SLAM system based on bionic eyes. *IEEE Trans. Med. Robot. Bionics* **2020**, *2*, 391–398. [CrossRef]
40. Hu, L.; Shen, C. A study of visual servo system based on binocular camera. In *Proceedings of the 5th International Conference on Electrical Engineering and Automatic Control*; Springer: Berlin/Heidelberg, Germany, 2016; pp. 1105–1112. [CrossRef]
41. Hu, P.; Hao, X.; Li, J.; Cheng, C.; Wang, A. Design and implementation of binocular vision system with an adjustable baseline and high synchronization. In Proceedings of the 2018 IEEE 3rd International Conference on Image, Vision and Computing (ICIVC), Chongqing, China, 27–29 June 2018; IEEE: New York, NY, USA, 2018; pp. 566–570. [CrossRef]
42. Xu, X.; Sun, Y.; Duan, H.; Deng, Y.; Zeng, Z. Maritime Target Saliency Detection for UAV Based on the Stimulation Competition Selection Mechanism of Raptor Vision. *Guid. Navig. Control.* **2023**, *3*, 2350012. [CrossRef]
43. Jia, H.; Li, S. Scene Analysis Based on Horse Vision System. In Proceedings of the MVA 2011 IAPR Conference on Machine Vision Applications, Nara, Japan, 13–15 June 2011; pp. 267–270.
44. Xu, Y.; Liu, C.; Cui, H.; Song, Y.; Yue, X.; Feng, L.; Wu, L. Environment Perception with Chameleon-Inspired Active Vision Based on Shifty Behavior for WMRs. *Appl. Sci.* **2023**, *13*, 6069. [CrossRef]
45. Wang, B.; Zhang, B.; Yu, D. The Bionic Research on Avian Visual Structure in Multi-Target Monitoring. In Proceedings of the 5th International Conference on Advanced Design and Manufacturing Engineering, Shenzhen, China, 19–20 September 2015; Atlantis Press: Paris, France, 2015; pp. 340–346. [CrossRef]
46. Bogatyreva, O.; Shillerov, A.; Bogatyrev, N. Patterns in TRIZ contradiction matrix: Integrated and distributed systems. In Proceedings of the 4th ETRIA Symposium, Florence, Italy, 3–5 November 2004; pp. 35–42.
47. Batemanazan, V.; Jaafar, A.; Kadir, R.A.; Nayan, N.M. Improving usability with TRIZ: A review. In Proceedings of the Advances in Visual Informatics: 5th International Visual Informatics Conference, IVIC 2017, Bangi, Malaysia, 28–30 November 2017; Proceedings 5; Springer: Berlin/Heidelberg, Germany, 2017; pp. 625–635. [CrossRef]
48. Lv, B.; Xue, Z.; Wei, H.; Li, Y. Exploration of Design Methods Based on Bionic Functional Modules. In *Journal of Physics: Conference Series*; IOP Publishing: Bristol, UK 2021; Volume 1939, p. 012078. [CrossRef]

49. Yongquan, Y.; Ying, H.; Minghui, W. The related matter-elements in extension detecting and application. In Proceedings of the Third International Conference on Information Technology and Applications (ICITA'05), Sydney, Australia, 4–7 July 2005; IEEE New York, NY, USA, 2005; Volume 1, pp. 411–414. [CrossRef]
50. Jones, M.P.; Pierce, K.E., Jr.; Ward, D. Avian vision: A review of form and function with special consideration to birds of prey *J. Exot. Pet Med.* **2007**, *16*, 69–87. [CrossRef]
51. Pettigrew, J.D. Evolution of Binocular Vision. In *Visual Neuroscience*; Cambridge University Press: Cambridge, UK, 1986 pp. 208–222, ISBN 0521258294.
52. McComb, D.; Tricas, T.; Kajiura, S. Enhanced visual fields in hammerhead sharks. *J. Exp. Biol.* **2009**, *212*, 4010–4018. [CrossRef] [PubMed]
53. Clarke, P.; Whitteridge, D. The projection of the retina, including the 'red area', on to the optic tectum of the pigeon. *Q. J. Exp. Physiol. Cogn. Med. Sci. Transl. Integr.* **1976**, *61*, 351–358. [CrossRef]
54. O'Rourke, C.T.; Hall, M.I.; Pitlik, T.; Fernández-Juricic, E. Hawk eyes I: Diurnal raptors differ in visual fields and degree of eye movement. *PLoS ONE* **2010**, *5*, e12802. [CrossRef]
55. Gregory-Evans, C.Y.; Gregory-Evans, K. Foveal hypoplasia: The case for arrested development. *Expert Rev. Ophthalmol.* **2011**, *6*, 565–574. [CrossRef]
56. Fite, K.V.; Lister, B.C. Bifoveal vision in Anolis lizards. *Brain, Behav. Evol.* **1981**, *19*, 144–154. [CrossRef] [PubMed]
57. Tucker, V.A. The deep fovea, sideways vision and spiral flight paths in raptors. *J. Exp. Biol.* **2000**, *203*, 3745–3754. [CrossRef] [PubMed]
58. Pettigrew, J.D.; Collin, S.P.; Ott, M. Convergence of specialised behaviour, eye movements and visual optics in the sandlance (Teleostei) and the chameleon (Reptilia). *Curr. Biol.* **1999**, *9*, 421–424. [CrossRef]
59. Land, M.F. Eye movements of vertebrates and their relation to eye form and function. *J. Comp. Physiol. A* **2015**, *201*, 195–214 [CrossRef] [PubMed]
60. Waldvogel, J.A. The bird's eye view. *Am. Sci.* **1990**, *78*, 342–353.
61. Tanner, J.; Itti, L. A top-down saliency model with goal relevance. *J. Vis.* **2019**, *19*, 11. [CrossRef]

applied sciences

MDPI

Article

Applied Mechatronic: A Sensor-Based Modification of an External Fixator According to Mitkovic

Vladimir Antić [1], Miodrag Manić [2], Milan Mitković [3], Nikola Korunović [2], Danijela Protić [1], Radomir Prodanović [1,*], Denis Kučević [4], Gordana Ostojić [5] and Stevan Stankovski [5]

[1] Center for Applied Mathematics and Electronics, 11000 Belgrade, Serbia; avladimir@ptt.rs (V.A.); danijelaprotic318@gmail.com (D.P.)
[2] Faculty of Mechanical Engineering, University of Nis, 18000 Nis, Serbia; miodrag.manic@masfak.ni.ac.rs (M.M.); korunovic.nikola@gmail.com (N.K.)
[3] Medical Faculty, University of Nis, 18000 Nis, Serbia; milanmitkovic@hotmail.com
[4] Faculty of Agriculture, University of Novi Sad, 21000 Novi Sad, Serbia; denis.kucevic@stocarstvo.edu.rs
[5] Center for Identification Technology, Faculty of Technical Sciences, University of Novi Sad, 21000 Novi Sad, Serbia; goca@uns.ac.rs (G.O.); stevan@uns.ac.rs (S.S.)
* Correspondence: radomir.prodanovic@vs.rs

Abstract: External fixators are frequently used to treat complex fractures with multiple bone fragments and soft tissue injuries. Inaccurate assessment of bone union and premature removal of the fixator may necessitate revisions and prolong treatment. The decision to remove an external fixator typically depends on an orthopedist's experience. The accuracy of diagnosis can be improved by using a force sensor integrated into the modified external fixator according to Mitkovic. A sensor measuring axial compressive force is mounted between two vertical rods. Experiments with the modified external fixator were carried out using three different axial loads delivered by the universal electromechanical testing machine (UETM) and a sensor that detected the corresponding axial force. Springs with variable rigidity were used to simulate bone callus stiffness. Low rigidity springs represented a high elasticity callus, whereas high rigidity springs represented a callus with lower elasticity. The results show that the force detected by the sensor was nearly identical to the force delivered by the UETM while the callus did not form, decreased as spring rigidity increased, and eventually zeroed out as the leg healed. The findings indicated that using modified external fixator according to Mitkovic can help orthopedists assess bone healing more accurately.

Keywords: bone healing; external fixation; sensors; wireless transmission; axial load measurement; increased precision

1. Introduction

A bone fracture can be partial or complete and is usually caused by a fall from a height, accident, osteoporosis, and overuse [1]. In [2], the authors describe four phases of secondary bone fracture healing: hematoma formation (1–2 weeks), granulation tissue formation (2–4 weeks), bone callus formation (4–8 weeks), and bone remodeling (8–12+ weeks). Callus is the new bone tissue formed at the fracture site. It is elastic and hardens over time, reaching the stiffness of healthy bones by the end of healing. The callus deflection is greatest at the beginning and the lowest at the end of healing, when it is equivalent to the deflection of a healthy bone.

The bone healing process requires a short distance between fracture fragments with very small freedom of movement until new bone tissue develops. Until the twentieth century, immobilization was the primary technique to hold bone fragments in place. Bone fixation implants emerged with the development of medicine. There are two types of severe bone fracture fixation. Internal fixation involves inserting the entire fixation implant under the skin, while external fixation uses pins inserted into the bone, passed through the soft tissues and skin, and attached to a frame outside the body [3]. Discomfort and possible pin tract infection are considered disadvantages of external fixation [4]. An external fixator, according to Mitkovic, is a minimally invasive 3D fixation system typically used to treat open fractures with a higher risk of infection, complex fractures, and fractures with severe trauma of the surrounding nerves and blood vessels [5]. It consists of bars, adjustable clamps, and clamp-carriers designed to be highly adaptable to different fracture fragments position.

Long bones fractures (femur, tibia, etc.) are the most common types of injuries that, in addition to expected discomfort, can lead to reduced or lost limb function [6–8] and, also, to complications such as deep infection, vascular or nerve damage [9], delayed union, malunion, and nonunion [10–13]. Delayed union occurs when bone does not heal at the expected rate, malunion is followed by bone healing but not in the proper position, whereas nonunion occurs when broken fragments fail to be connected by the new bone [10]. The authors of [11] conducted a study on the rate and predictions of patient readmission for surgical treatment due to bone healing complications (8% of patients were readmitted to the hospital). In [12], the authors found that vulnerability of the soft tissues surrounding the fracture increases the susceptibility to non-union and infection. The authors of [13] discuss a morbidity associated with a long bone nonunion. In addition, several studies [14–17] discuss emergency fracture care in cattle orthopedics. The authors of [14,15,17] discuss external skeletal fixation (ESF) as a rigid immobilization, while the author of [16] discusses long bone fractures complications. However, the external fixation on the cattle is outside of the scope of this study.

Integration of a sensor technology into the external fixator is a strategy that provides a more accurate decision on bone healing. A modified external fixator according to Mitkovic is an electrically active system in which force is detected by a sensor integrated into the existing structure [18]. At the beginning of the treatment, the sensor readings correspond to half of the patient's weight, implying that the broken leg was not loaded. When the callus hardens, the sensor deflection changes due to the axial load. As the force in the leg increases the force detected by the sensor drops to near-zero levels.

In the experiments, three different axial loads delivered by the Shimadzu universal electromechanical testing machine (UETM) (50 N, 250 N, and 500 N) are compared with axial forces detected by the sensor, with three springs of different rigidity ($k = 1.5$ N/mm, $k = 3.8$ N/mm, and $k = 7.5$ N/mm) used to simulate different stages of callus hardening [2]. The results show that the force detected by the sensor was almost identical to the force delivered by the UETM ($k = 0$ N/mm) and decreased as the spring rigidity increased. When the patient fully recovers, the sensor detects only minor elastic deformation caused by deflection of the bone and weight of fixator parts located above the sensor.

From a technical perspective, the fixator may be removed when sensor reading approaches zero. However, from a medical perspective, the choice to remove the fixator is influenced by the orthopedist's subjective assessment. The results of this research indicate that the functional upgrades to the external fixator according to Mitkovic corroborate the evaluations made by orthopedists. An objective approach to using data from the sensor can facilitate clinical decision-making. It is important to highlight that the findings discussed in this article are based on mechanical tests, with plans for clinical trials to be carried out in the future.

2. Related Work

External fixator systems are characterized by their simplicity and versatility of use, ability to reduce soft-tissue damage, stability at the bone screw interface, and rigidity [19]. The decision to remove an external fixator is typically based on the interpretation of clinical results and the experience of an orthopedist. In [20] the authors discuss the lack of standardized methods for assessing bone union that result in significant disagreements among orthopedists in both clinical practice and research. Currently, X-rays and magnetic resonance imaging are the primary but unsafe diagnostic tool used to assess the callus formation and the mechanical stability of the bone. Other clinical evaluation parameters assessed by the orthopedist include the pain, soft tissue healing, (in)stability of the patient, and weight bearing [21]. In addition, mechanical assessment tools can be used to decide about the stiffness of the callus from the early stages of its formation until complete union. Direct methods (i.e., assessing the fracture stiffness by measuring the deflection at the fracture site) have the major disadvantage of removing the external fixator for each measurement. Indirect approaches (i.e., measuring strain via external fixation) have been more extensively applied. However, only a few studies have examined the displacement of external fixator components as a mean of monitoring the fracture healing.

In [22] the authors present design of a dynamic external fixator system used to treat open tibial fractures. It consists of an inner rod with axial motion in the outer tube for dynamization to improve bone healing. Clamps for rods and tube provide six degrees of freedom. An open clamp is designed to limit tube movement. Distal nuts are used for bone gap closure function. This design is developed based on the benefits of dynamization (a gradually decreasing construct-stability of a fixator as a therapy used for the final phase of fracture healing), increased union rate and the simplicity of mono-lateral frame. It is simple to use, safe, and provide a stable structure in which rigidity and alignment can be adjusted as needed during the treatment. In [23], the authors describe three-step dynamization of the hexapod circular external fixator that is primary based on the experience of an orthopedist, with no set criteria. The first step is to loosen two struts arbitrarily, then remove the loosened struts, and finally remove the remaining struts one at a time. The authors of [24] propose a non-invasive method based on changes in stress transmission, the location of stress-sensitive points, and the displacement in an external fixator system during healing process of tibial fractures. Their research focuses on developing finite element models for fractures treated with unilateral external fixation. The intersections of the lowest screw and the bone cortex, as well as the second screw and the connecting rod, can be used as sensitive points for monitoring the healing. As a next research step, the authors propose investigating the feasibility of placing non-invasive, compact sensors on external fixators. This can assist orthopedists to accurately assess fracture healing, allowing for more informed treatment decisions, including removal of the external fixator.

The orthopedist can remove the vertical rod of the fixator to check the bone healing process. If the pain persists during the orthopedist's manual pressure at both sides of the fixator, the vertical rod should be reinserted into the device and treatment should be continued. To facilitate the assessment of the callus hardening without requiring numerous X-ray images, we have modified an external fixator according to Mitkovic [25] that detects micromovements between bone fragments and have provided data on callus elasticity based on sensor readings.

3. Modified External Fixator According to Mitkovic

In [25], the authors describe an external fixator according to Mitkovic as an external fixator that allows for gradual reduction in fixation stiffness and leads to a high rate of successful healing. The fracture fixation device facilitates the achievements of a balanced

3D wedge configuration at an angle of 90°, as well as at any other desired angle [26]. This design represents the simplest concept of external fixation, consisting of a road, clamp carriers, clamps, and pins, which can be interconnected in various configurations to form frames suitable for all trauma care requirements, primarily those that are complex and have associated soft tissue damage [27,28]. An external fixator according to Mitkovic is shown in Figure 1a. However, despite the fact that this fixator has a number of benefits, precise indicators for its removal have yet to be properly established [18]. The modified external fixator according to Mitkovic is shown in Figure 1b.

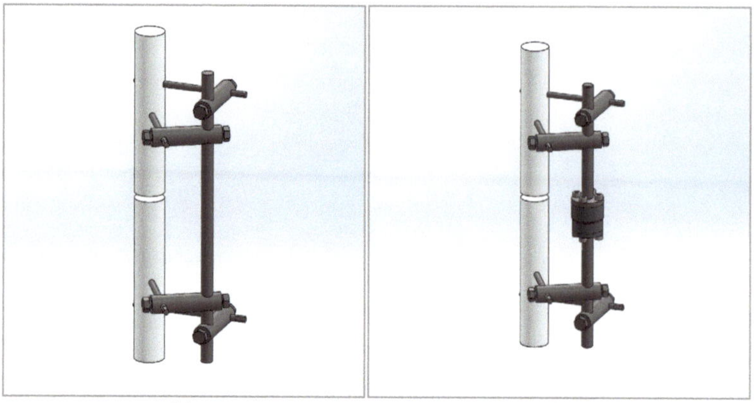

(a) (b)

Figure 1. External fixators: (**a**) external fixator according to Mitkovic; (**b**) modified external fixator according to Mitkovic.

The sensor is a cylinder with threaded holes on both its upper and lower surfaces, built-in between two vertical rods connecting the upper and lower parts of the supporting structure. The measuring unit is a steel loaded element with mounted strain gages. Flanges are attached to the ends of the rods and are connected to the upper and lower sides of the sensor. With this design, there is no need to loosen the screws in the clamps fixing the parts of the vertical rod during the recovery period. The disadvantage of the design is that it does not prevent the sensor from being loaded by a bending moment resulting from eccentric action of axial comprehensive force. The alternative that best fits the experimental settings is the bending moment determined by the patient's weight. A sensor capable of measuring forces up to 10 kN (~1000 kg weight) can withstand a bending moment of 120 Nm. The compressive axial loads are related to the distances between two parts of the fractured bone. The sensor unit can be easily integrated with the external fixator and used to distinguish the external wedges relative displacements to provide information on the callus stiffness, determined as follows:

$$\text{stiffness} = \frac{F}{d}, \tag{1}$$

where d represents the displacement and F represents the force exerted through the leg.

For the purpose of this research, the U93A force sensor is used to detect small changes in force and to convert mechanical stimuli into an electrical signal, in response to the force exerted trough the leg [18]. The sensor dimensions are $\Phi 35 \times 30$. It has four M5 threaded holes on the upper and lower surfaces. The U93A models with 0–10 V or 4–20 mA configurations are available, as well as a digital module featuring an I/O-link interface. A significant feature of this sensor is the 0.05 mm deflection at the full load.

Since the sensor does not measure force directly but detects it through deflection, calibration is performed before use, through the manufacturer's application. When an axial load is applied, the measurement body deforms, which leads to strain near the strain gages. These gages are configured to create a Wheatstone bridge circuit, generating an output signal proportional to the variation in resistance and, consequently, the magnitude of the force, when it is under voltage. The relationship between the force F [N] and the sensor sensitivity S [mV/V] is linear ($F = k \cdot S$). The calibration factor k is determined by manufacturer based on two reference points: the origin and the maximum nominal load of 10 kN, which corresponds to a generated electrical signal of 1.2144 mV/V (Figure 2).

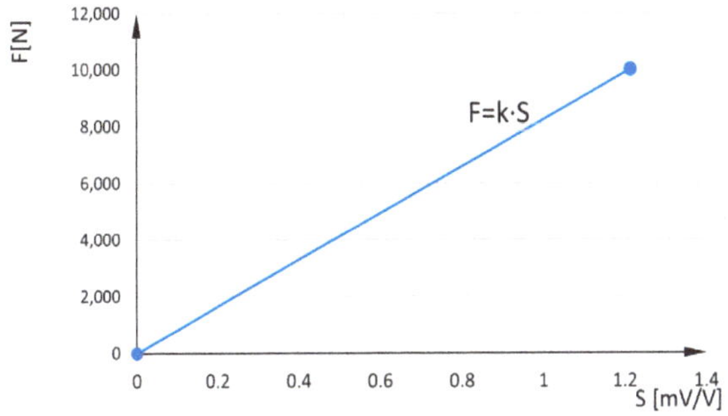

Figure 2. Relation between axial force and sensor sensitivity.

The sensor is connected to a smartphone or tablet via Bluetooth and a free app, allowing measurement results to be displayed and recorded for future data analysis. The communication module is connected to the sensor via cable and has its own power supply (it is also power supply for the sensor).

A Mantracourt B24-SSBC-A (B24) is used for wireless transmission between the sensor and a mobile device. The B24 telemetry strain bridge sensor transmitter is designed to provide measurement systems with user-friendly access (C style enclosure with integrated battery). It enables strain measurements at close range allowing immediate engagement with data and projects. Effective power electronic provides high input sensitivity of ±6 mV/V, ±12 mV/V, ±24 mV/V, and ±48 mV/V. It aims to work for up to 3 months of continuous use of three samples per second for a close range up to 90 m, and ideally up to 12 transmitters by a single device. The transmission rate is adjustable from 10 times/second to once per 10 s. The B24 can be calibrated in kilograms and other weight units such as tons or pounds. The B24 iOS and Android App for B24 Bluetooth Transmitter interface (B24 App) generate dashboards for hands-on measurements, and display data from the strain bridge module directly on Android or iOS. In addition, the B24 App creates real-time measuring projects and can select 5 different tiles to customize dashboard. Data can be expressed as mathematical equations to describe exactly what is displayed. The B24.NET Driver Pack contains. NET drivers for configuring and calibrating B24 modules from a PC.

4. Experimental Results

The experiments were carried out in March and April 2025, at the Faculty of Mechanical Engineering, University of Nis. The objective of the experiments was to analyze the design and operational aspects of the modified fixator as a means for qualitatively assessing the healing of fractured bones.

4.1. Experiment Setup

The experiments are conducted on a fixator equipped with a U93A sensor. A sensor design sensor includes flanges that precisely match the sensor's upper and lower surfaces. The connection is secured with four M5 screws to replicate real-world conditions; the rod and sensor are fixed until the end of the treatment.

The Shimadzu computer-controlled UETM is used to measure the compressive axial load. The UETM with the sensor inserted between joints for compression tests is shown in Figure 3a. Sensor inserted in the middle of the vertical rod is shown in Figure 3b.

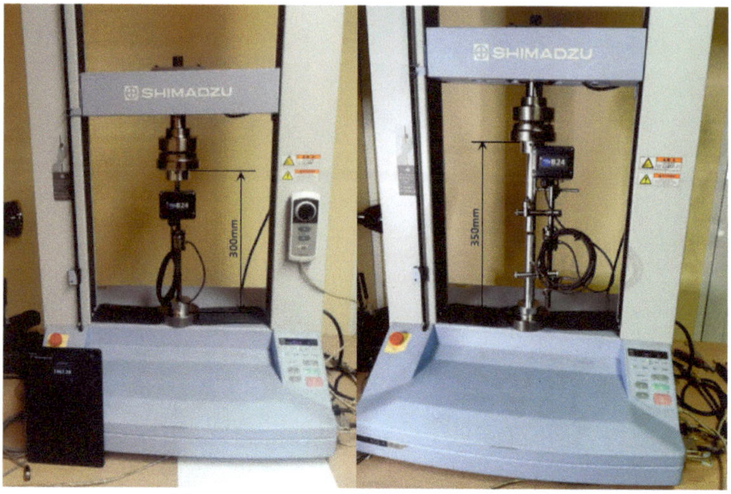

(a) (b)

Figure 3. Experimental setup for testing the modified external fixator according to Mitkovic. (**a**) The sensor is inserted between the joints of UETM. (**b**) The sensor is integrated in the middle of the vertical rod.

UETM is suitable for extensive testing of metallic and non-metallic materials in tension, compression, bending, torsion, friction, peel, adhesion, and penetration. The stress and strain are easily controllable with a Jog controller that allows hand-held control of the crosshead position. The Jog dial makes fine positioning easy. A built-in main operational panel enables the development and storing of test conditions, allowing testing without having to connect to the PC. The UETM comes with the industry-leading TRAPEZIUM X data processing software, which offers an unrivaled level of performance and provides improved productivity and efficiency for quality control operations. Since TRAPEZIUM X and the B24 App enable data recording and processing, it is possible to confirm that modified external fixator according to Mitkovic provides better monitoring of bone recovery processes. In qualitatively superior level, the bone union process is monitored and the moment when the use of the fixator is unnecessary is determined (i.e., fixator removing).

4.2. Measurements of Axial Loads

When a bone breaks, the body begins to form an elastic callus to heal the fracture. The callus hardens over time, reaching the stiffness of healthy bone by the end of recovery. The bone callus stiffness is simulated by springs of various rigidity: k = 0 N/mm, k = 1.5 N/mm, k = 3.8 N/mm, and k = 7.5 N/mm, which correspond to the four phases of secondary healing [2]. More detailed explanations can be found in [29–32]. To limit variability in geometry and mechanical properties, two 25 mm diameter aluminum rods are used to simulate a broken bone and injured tissues. Because stiffness and elasticity are inversely proportional, a low rigidity spring simulates a high elasticity callus during the early stages of bone union. A high rigidity spring simulates the callus with reduced elasticity and increased stiffness. Bonded connections are used to simulate the joints between the elements of the fixator.

Since no medical data on the load level applied to the external fixator according to Mitkovic was available, the UETM was used to deliver loads by increasing compressive axial force from 0 to 300 N and then decreasing it back to 0 N every 0.5 s. Small variations in forces delivered by UETM and measured by the sensor were detected (See Figure 4).

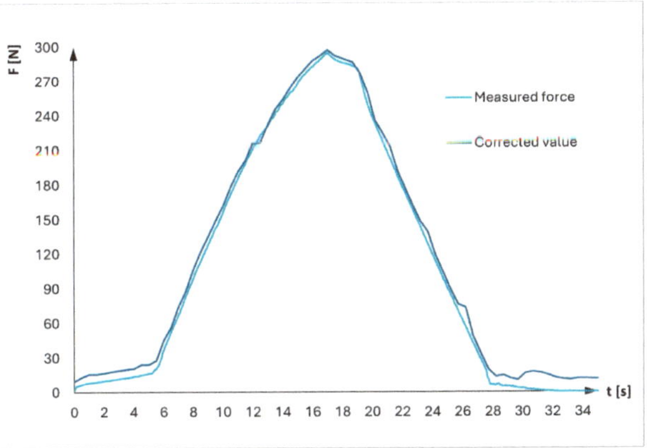

Figure 4. Correction of force generated by UETM.

The accuracy of the UETM control software was verified at the very beginning to minimize measurement errors when comparing the force exerted by the UETM with the force detected by the sensor placed between its joints (Figure 3a). The sensor reading served as a reference point. The result indicated that the force delivered by the UETM was slightly higher than the reference value. A correction factor of 1.0164 was determined by comparing these values. Therefore, the force values delivered by the UETM were adjusted by dividing them by this correction factor during experiments.

4.3. *Experiments on Modified External Fixator According to Mitkovic*

Experiments with the modified external fixator are conducted using three different axial loads delivered by the UETM (50 N, 250 N, and 500 N), which corresponds to the patient's ability to tolerate pressure in the injured leg until the onset of pain. When leaning feet, the patient slowly alternates between loading the bones of healthy and injured leg. The value of this load ranges from zero, when the foot has no contact with the ground, up to its maximum when foot bears the entire weight of the body.

The simulation of slow leaning towards the feet is performed by gradually applying three forces delivered by the UETM at 0.5 s intervals, ranging from 0 to 50 N, 250 N, or 500 N, and then returning to zero. Different callus stiffnesses are estimated by measuring for each spring, including one without a spring. Each measurement is conducted twice, resulting in a total of 24 experiments.

Figures 5–7 show a comparative view of forces that load the fixator, which are delivered by the UETM and represent the weight of the patient, as well as values of the forces measured by the sensor at different loads and different rigidity of the springs (12 measurements in total).

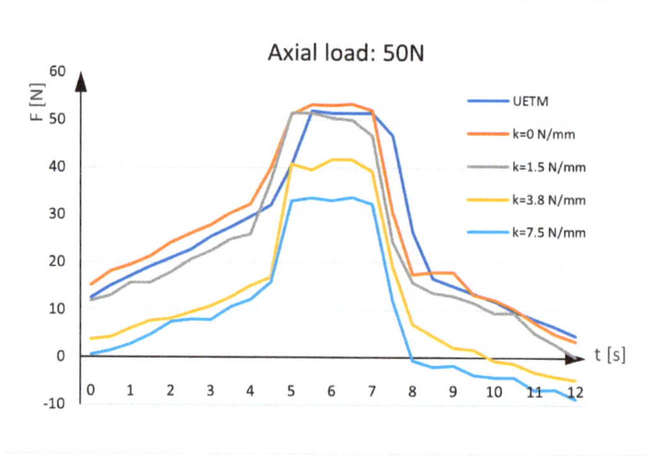

Figure 5. Sensor measurements. UETM load: 50N.

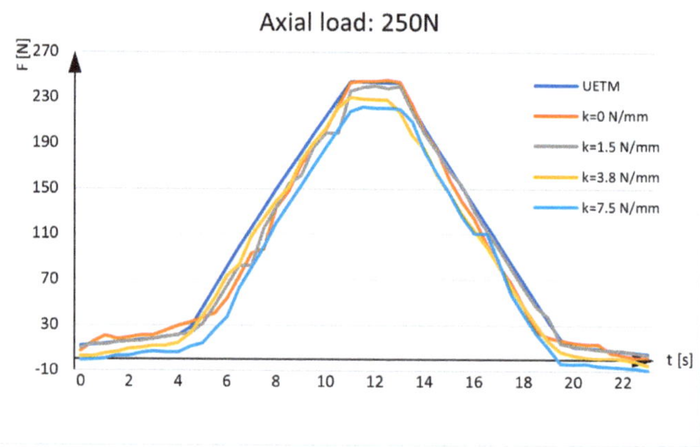

Figure 6. Sensor measurements. UETM load: 250N.

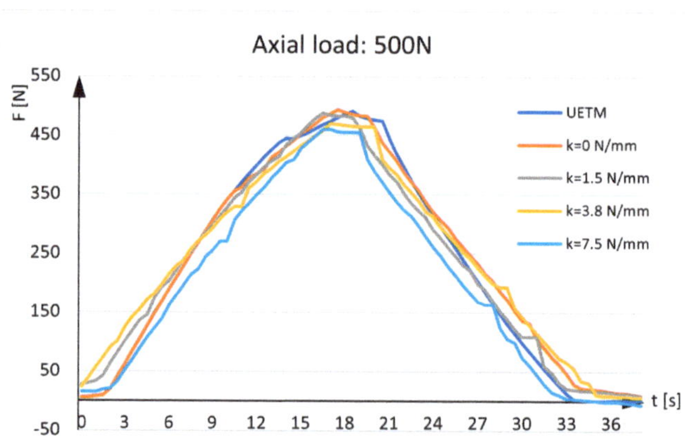

Figure 7. Sensor measurements. UETM load: 500N.

The diagrams given in the figures have the same shapes and imply that force measured by the sensor is almost identical to the force delivered by the UETM when k = 0 N/mm. The diagrams change due to the different load values delivered by the UETM, the different time periods required to increase and decrease the force from zero to its maximum value, and rigidity of springs. It should be noted that, when the springs are positioned between the aluminum rods, they are under strain, and forces measured by the sensor deviate from the forces delivered by the UETM, which rise with spring rigidity. As the spring returns to its neutral position, it pulls the rods aside, delivering load transfers to the sensor and resulting in tensile stress. Because the sensor tends to elongate, the force values represented in the diagrams tend to show negative values.

Figure 8 shows the measurement in real situations. The results depict a patient's gradual leaning on the injured leg until the leg bears half a weight (the patient's weight is evenly distributed on both legs). As load-bearing capacity improves, the force measured by the sensor decreases. A horizontal line represents half of the patient's weight.

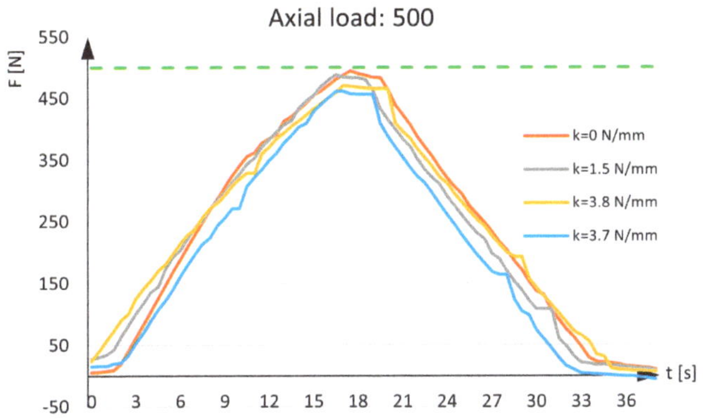

Figure 8. Axial load: 500N. The green line represents the maximum weight of one leg.

Figure 8 also depicts recovery with the curvilinear lines, representing the force detected by the sensor. The curves are distinct from the horizontal line and approach the x-axis ($y = 0$). When the patient fully recovers, the sensor recording will not be zero because the bone will always have minor elastic deformation, there are axial deflection of the bone, and there will be an influence from the weight of fixator parts located above the sensor.

4.4. Discussion

The diagrams displaying the results of force measurement without springs show that the force values delivered by the UETM and measured by the sensor are nearly identical. Certain variations are caused by elastic deformations of the fixator parts connecting to the aluminum rods and the sensor itself, as well as the pins, clamps, and the upper and lower vertical rods. Moreover, the rods and the sensor are subjected to complex stresses that include both axial pressure and bending.

Force measurements with springs are more realistic, since they take into account callus hardening through the recovery period. The diagrams illustrate that the values of the forces measured by the sensor are smaller than the values of the forces delivered by the UETM, with the difference increasing as spring rigidities increase. These deviations are expected and desirable since, from a medical standpoint, they indicate callus hardening.

There are no established diagnostic criteria at this point of the research to evaluate sensor data concerning a clinical threshold that would convert sensor data into practical decisions and provide objective measurements. The interpretation of these data still depends on the orthopedist's experience. Further evaluation of sensor-based external fixation is necessary before it can be widely used in clinical practice.

5. Conclusions and Further Work

Classical diagnostic approaches for determining full recovery after a long bone fracture do not provide precise information about whether the bone has healed completely. The assessment on fixator removal is mostly based on orthopedist's experience and X-ray images. Occasionally, after diagnostic tests indicated the healing process was supposed to be completed and the fixator should be removed, patients return to hospital because of discomfort, pain, and/or infection. A modified external fixator, according to Mitkovic, provides the orthopedist with accurate data based on sensor measurements of change in the compressive force.

Experiments with the modified external fixator were carried out using three distinct axial loads delivered by the UETM, which simulated patient's ability to lean to the leg until pain occurred, and a sensor that measured the resulting force. Springs of varying rigidity were used to imitate bone callus stiffness. Low rigidity springs depicted a high elasticity callus, whereas high rigidity springs replicated a callus with reduced elasticity and increased stiffness. The results showed that the force detected by the sensor was nearly identical to the force delivered by the UETM for k = 0 N/mm and decreased as spring rigidity increased.

As the next research step, the modified external fixator according to Mitkovic is planned to be used in the clinical practice of medical co-authors in real-world situations.

Furthermore, the modified external fixator is planned to be upgraded with communication equipment for remote data transmission of axial load measurements. Remote transmission eliminates the need for the orthopedist and the patient to be present at the same place during periodic check-ups. The benefits to the patient include enhanced comfort, reduced stress and a variety of others. The results on bending and axial compressive force over time provide information on the dynamics of callus hardening. These data can be used to build machine learning models, which could predict the patient's recovery time. In this way, it would be possible, for example, to estimate the costs of treatment, absenteeism from the workplace due to injury, and so forth. Artificial intelligence algorithms can also be used for data processing and decision-making. Given data can be integrated with digital health platforms to facilitate remote monitoring and data sharing. Data analysis could be later used for different medical applications. It is important to note that processing and transmitting personal data necessitate data protection, which implies the use of cryptographic algorithms.

In some severe cases, where the bone must be stretched, a relative gradual axial separation of bone parts over time intervals with a distance proportional to the bone union may be performed. This can be accomplished by using screws built into the modified fixator to transform rotational movement into a rectilinear one. The screw can be tuned by orthopedist or automatically using a small, sensitive stepper motor actuator (SMA) at a specified angle to separate bone parts dependent on the angle of rotation and the step of the coil. SMA consists of a synchronous stepper motor that moves in discrete steps, a mechanical transmission mechanism that converts the motor's rotary motion into the linear motion, and a control system that manages the stepper motor operations. The communications protocols used to control stepper motors are IEEE 802.x, TCP/IP, and UDP. SMA control can be implemented using a variety of microcontroller chips with Wi-Fi interfaces, such as Microchip PIC16F (Microchip Technology, Chandler, Arizona, USA) and Espressif System ESP 8266 (Espressif Systems, Shanghai, China).

Last but not least, there is some possibility for using the modified external fixator on cattle's long bones to improve clinical management of selected fractures. However, it should be kept in mind that this structure should be customized to the specific use on livestock.

Author Contributions: Conceptualization, V.A., R.P., M.M. (Miodrag Manić), M.M. (Milan Mitković) and D.P.; methodology, V.A., M.M. (Miodrag Manić), N.K. and M.M. (Milan Mitković); validation, M.M. (Miodrag Manić), R.P., D.P. and M.M. (Milan Mitković); formal analysis, G.O., S.S., M.M. (Miodrag Manić), M.M. (Milan Mitković), N.K. and D.K.; investigation, V.A., N.K. and D.P.; resources, S.S., G.O. and M.M. (Miodrag Manić); data curation, D.K., M.M. (Miodrag Manić) and R.P.; visualization: D.P., V.A., R.P. and N.K.; writing—original draft preparation, V.A., D.P., R.P., M.M. (Miodrag Manić), M.M. (Milan Mitković), G.O., S.S. and D.K.; writing—review and editing V.A., D.P., R.P., M.M. (Miodrag Manić), M.M. (Milan Mitković), G.O., S.S. and D.K.; supervision, M.M. (Miodrag Manić), M.M. (Milan Mitković) and S.S.; funding acquisition, G.O., S.S. and D.K. All authors have read and agreed to the published version of the manuscript.

Funding: This research was funded by the Provincial Secretariat for Higher Education and Scientific Research of Autonomous Province of Vojvodina, Serbia, through project (contract number 003077303 2024 09418 003 000 000 001/2).

Institutional Review Board Statement: Not applicable.

Informed Consent Statement: Not applicable.

Data Availability Statement: Dataset available on request from the authors.

Acknowledgments: The authors thank the Provincial Secretariat for Higher Education and Scientific Research of Autonomous Province of Vojvodina, Republic of Serbia.

Conflicts of Interest: The authors declare no conflicts of interest.

References

1. Court-Brown, C.M.; Bugler, K.E.; Clement, N.D.; Duckworth, N.D.; McQueen, M.M. The epidemiology of open fractures in adults. A 15-year review. *Injury* **2012**, *43*, 891–897. [CrossRef] [PubMed]
2. Sheen, J.R.; Mabrouk, A.; Garla, V.V. Fracture healing overview. In *National Library of Medicine*; StatPearls Publishing: Treasure Island, FL, USA, 2023. Available online: https://www.ncbi.nlm.nih.gov/books/NBK551678/ (accessed on 13 May 2025).
3. Fernando, P.L.N.; Abeygunawanardane, A.; Wijesinghe, P.C.I.; Dharmartne, P.; Silva, P. An engineering review of external fixators. *Med. Eng. Phys.* **2021**, *98*, 91–103. [CrossRef]
4. Hoenig, M.; Gao, F.; Kinder, J.; Zhang, L.Q.; Collinge, C.; Merk, B.R. Extra-articular distal tibia fractures: A mechanical evaluation of 4 different treatment methods. *J. Othopedic Trauma* **2010**, *24*, 30–35. [CrossRef]
5. Mitkovic, M.B.; Bumbasirevic, M.; Golubovic, Z.; Micic, I.; Mladenovic, D.; Milenkovic, S.; Lesic, A.; Bumbasirevic, V.; Pavlovic, P.; Karalejic, S.; et al. New concept in external fixation. *Acta Chir. Jugosl.* **2005**, *52*, 107–111. [CrossRef] [PubMed]
6. Cordelle, M.Z.; Snelling, S.J.; Mouthuy, P.A. Skeletal muscle tissue engineering: From tissue regeneration to biorobotics. *Cyborg Bionic Syst.* **2025**, *6*, 0279. [CrossRef]
7. Court-Brown, C.M.; Rimmer, S.; Parkash, U.; McQueen, M.M. The epidemiology of open long bone fractures. *Injury* **1998**, *29*, 529–534. [CrossRef]
8. Bisaccia, M.; Cappiello, A.; Meccariello, A.; Meccariello, L.; Rinonapoli, G.; Falzarano, G.; Medici, A.; Ibaney Vicente, C.; Piscitelli, L.; Stano, V.; et al. Nail or plate in the management of distal extra-articular tibial fractures, what is better? Valutation of outcomes. *SICOT-J* **2018**, *4*, 2. [CrossRef]
9. Gai, Y.; Yin, Y.; Guan, L.; Zhang, S.; Chen, J.; Yang, J.; Zhou, H.; Li, J. Rational design of bioactive materials for bone hemostasis and defect repair. *Cyborg Bionic Syst.* **2023**, *4*, 0058. [CrossRef]
10. Schindler, C.R.; Mazi, I. Long bone fractures. In *Acute Care Surgery in Geriatric Patients*; Petrone, P., Bratwaite, C.E., Eds.; Springer: Cham, Switzerland, 2023; pp. 241–251. [CrossRef]
11. Ekegren, C.L.; Edwards, E.R.; De Steiger, R.; Gabbe, B.J. Incidence, cost and predictors of non-union, delayed union and mal-union following long bone fracture. *Int. J. Environ. Res. Public Health* **2018**, *15*, 2845. [CrossRef]

12. Noorlander-Borgdorff, M.P.; Sekercan, A.; Young-Afat, D.A.; Bouman, M.; Botman, M.; Ginnakkopoulos, G.F. Nationwide study on open tibial fractures in the Netherlands: Incidence, demographics and level of hospital care. *Injury* **2024**, *55*, 111487. [CrossRef]
13. Nicholson, J.A.; Makaram, N.; Simpson, A.H.R.W.; Keating, J.F. Fracture nonunion in long bones: A literature review of risk factors and surgical management. *Injury* **2021**, *52*, S3–S11. [CrossRef]
14. Adams, S. The role of external fixation and emergency fracture management in bovine orthopedics. *Vet. Clin. N. Am. Food Anim Pract.* **1985**, *1*, 109–129. [CrossRef]
15. Vogel, S.; Anderson, D. External skeletal fixation of fractures in Cattle. *Vet. Clin. N. Am. Food Anim. Pract.* **2014**, *30*, 127–142 [CrossRef] [PubMed]
16. Irvine-Smith, G. External skeletal fixation. Presented at the World Small Animal Veterinary Association World Congress Proceedings, Cape Town, South Africa, 16–19 September 2014.
17. Sellahewa, T.; Weerashinghe, C.; Silva, P. Biomechanical evaluation method to optimize external fixator configuring in long bone fractures—Conceptual model and experimental validation using pilot study. *Appl. Sci.* **2021**, *11*, 8481. [CrossRef]
18. Antic, V.; Misic, D.; Manic, M. Strain sensor-based monitoring of smart orthopedic devices in lower limb fracture healing: A review. *Innov. Mech. Eng.* **2023**, *2*, 17–41.
19. Kouassi, K.J.E.; Cartiaux, O.; Fonokue, L.; Detrembleur, C.; Cornu, O. Biomechanical study of a low-cost external fixator for diaphyseal fractures of long bones. *J. Orthop. Surg. Res.* **2020**, *15*, 247. [CrossRef] [PubMed]
20. Cunningham, B.P.; Brazina, S.; Morshed, S.; Miclau, T. Fracture healing: A review of clinical, imaging and laboratory diagnostic options. *Injury* **2017**, *48*, 69–75. [CrossRef]
21. Sorriento, A.; Chiurazzi, M.; Fabbri, L.; Scaglione, M.; Dario, P.; Ciuti, G. A novel capacitive measurement device for longitudinal monitoring of bone fracture healing. *Sensors* **2021**, *21*, 6694. [CrossRef]
22. Suksathien, Y.; Suksathien, R. Clinical study of a new design multifunction dynamic external fixation system for open tibial fracture. *J. Med. Assoc. Thail.* **2011**, *94*, 1084–1088.
23. Mao, Y.; Lin, Q.; Yang, Q. The relation between the dynamization of hexapod circular external fixator and tibial mechanical properties. *Orthop. Surg.* **2023**, *15*, 1677–1684. [CrossRef]
24. Jia, X.; Shen, C.; Luo, B.; Yang, Y.; Zhang, K.; Deng, Y.; Wen, J.; Ma, L. How does the stress in the fixation device change during different stages of bone healing in the treatment of fractures? A finite element study of external fixation for tibial fractures. *Orthop Surg.* **2024**, *16*, 2821–2833. [CrossRef]
25. Milenkovic, S.; Mitkovic, M.M.; Mitkovic, M. External fixation of segmental tibial shaft fractures. *Eur. J. Trauma Emerg. Surg.* **2020**, *46*, 1123–1127. [CrossRef]
26. Milenkovic, S.; Mitkovic, M.M. External fixation of extra-articular open tibial fractures. *Acta Fac. Medicae Naissensis* **2018**, *35*, 330–336. [CrossRef]
27. Mitkovic, M.B.; Bumbasirevic, M.; Lesic, A.; Golubivic, Z. Dynamic external fixation of comminuted intra-articular fractures of the distal tibia (type C pilon fractures). *Acta Orthop. Belg.* **2003**, *68*, 508–514.
28. Mitkovic, M. Primena Metode i Aparata po Mitkoviću. In *Spoljna Fiksacija Kod Preloma Tibije*; Srpska akademija nauka i umetnosti Ogranak u Nišu: Niš, Serbia, 2020; Available online: https://www.mitkovic.org/news/pdf/IZVODZASAJT.pdf (accessed on 17 May 2025).
29. Ghiasi, M.S.; Chen, J.E.; Rodrigez, E.K.; Vaziri, A.; Nazarian, A. Computational modeling of human bone fracture healing affected by different conditions of initial healing stage. *BMC Musculoskelet. Disord.* **2019**, *20*, 562. [CrossRef]
30. Liu, Y.; Cai, F.; Liu, K.; Zhang, X.; Li, H.; Fu, X.; Zhang, T.; Yusufu, A. Bony callus stiffness indirectly evaluated by the axial load-share ratio in vivo as a guide to removing a monoliteral external fixator safety. *Int. Orthop.* **2021**, *45*, 3015–3023. [CrossRef]
31. Steiner, M.; Claes, L.; Ignatius, A.; Simon, U.; Wehner, T. Numerical simulation of callus healing for optimization of fracture fixation stiffness. *PLoS ONE* **2014**, *9*, e101370. [CrossRef]
32. Burny, F.; Burny, W.; Donkerwolcke, M.; Behrens, M. Effect on callus development on the deformation of external fixation frames *Int. Orthop.* **2012**, *36*, 2577–2580. [CrossRef]

MDPI AG
Grosspeteranlage 5
4052 Basel
Switzerland
Tel.: +41 61 683 77 34

Applied Sciences Editorial Office
E-mail: applsci@mdpi.com
www.mdpi.com/journal/applsci

www.ingramcontent.com/pod-product-compliance
Lightning Source LLC
Chambersburg PA
CBHW041342210926
51850CB00013B/2959
9783725844036